# Cardamom Tea

## By Noora

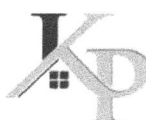

Serial Number: P2536240108
Title: Cardamom Tea
Author: Noora (Zahra) Mohammadiyoun
Layout: Merry Oskooei
Cover Designer & Character Illustration: Noora Mohammadiyoun
Portrait Cover Photographer: Shamin Zahabion
English editors: Mark McCready and Kevin Byrne
ISBN: 978-1-77892-249-7
Subject: Fiction, Memoir, Inspirational
Book format/Size: Paperback, A5
Pages: 116
Publication Date: July 2025
Publisher: Kidsocado Publishing House

Copyright © 2025 By Kidsocado Publishing House
All Rights Reserved, including the right of reproduction in whole or in part in any form.

## Kidsocado Publishing House
### Vancouver, Canada

Phone: +1 (236) 333-7248
WhatsApp: +1 (236) 333-7248
Email: info@kidsocado.com
Website: https://kidsocado.com
Address: 2100-1055 West Georgia St,
Vancouver, BC V6E 3P3, Canada

I have always wanted to be a source of pride for those who love me.

I dedicate this book to myself and to my God. Let this work stand as a radiant testament to my faith in Him.

To My Moonlight (Mahe Moniram)

my dear mother, whose unwavering encouragement has always been the spark behind my words. It was her joy that inspired me to sit, to write, and to see this book to completion.

To my beautiful family, my gifted yet unsung storytellers. May this book be the whisper that urges you to bring your own stories to life, to weave them into the next cherished book for the world to embrace.

With love, Noora :)

## About the Author

Zahra (Noora) Mohammadiyoun, the fourth and youngest child in a family of six, was born in Gonbad-e Kavus, a beautiful city in the northeast of Iran. Both of her parents were teachers. She spent her formative years studying various artistic disciplines in Mashhad, Gorgan, Qom, Tabriz, and Tehran. For many years, she has been serving as an honorary ambassador for the "SMA" (Spinal Muscular Atrophy) community in Iran and Turkey. Noora graduated with distinction in May 2023 and faced two unexpected challenges in 2024. She is a cheerful and eloquent individual with a spirit full of joy, creativity, and courage, who has created a new definition and image of faith, resilience, and endurance.

Noora is gifted not only in writing but also in art and graphic design.

She has something to say; just one encounter with her is enough to feel her passion for life. With that very love that flows through her being, she creates extraordinary pieces of art. She has also made a remarkable impact organizing cultural and social events in Vancouver. She is always striving to create warm spaces for dialogue, growth, unity, increased empathy, and uplifting group activities.

The book Cardamom Tea tells the story of Noora's journey through the unexpected darkness of life, guided by a powerful faith that blossomed in hardship and became her compass. Page by page, it carries the heartbeat of someone who chooses to live in gratitude: for hope, for the love of God, for existence itself, and for the beauty hidden in it all.

Life has never been easy , yet she believes it still holds countless wonders worth pursuing. For Noora, the longing to see her homeland, Iran, once again… to travel with her family, and to celebrate the gift of life, these became the beautiful reasons that kept her moving forward.

She recalls Sohrab's words: "As long as there are poppies, one must live." Yet she came to understand that life is not always so gentle. Even the poppies, like countless other things once cherished and lost, such as the beloved cheetah Pirooz[1], may fade away.

So perhaps it is more honest to say: "As long as the wheel of life keeps turning, so does our journey, and it is up to us to shape it. She knows it is difficult, yet she also believes it is possible." :)

---

1. Pirouz (Persian: پیروز , meaning victorious; 2022–2023) was the only surviving cub of the first Asiatic cheetahs born in captivity in Iran, gaining fame as one of the last of his kind.

**In the name of the Light that wraps the soul in mercy and brings life to every word:**

Writing has remarkable power; it feels like being in a classroom where you are both the student and the teacher. Sometimes you can surprise yourself with what comes out of your own mouth. making you proud of the student you've been because you've learned your lessons well and can convey them effectively.

The day I decided to write my story, an inner voice told me that my perspective and how I had navigated through all the sudden heavy experiences that happened could inspire many. This voice grew more confident as it said, "I will write it." so I placed my hands on the keyboard and began. It turned out to be harder than I had imagined.

It always seems that as we move forward in life, we expect things to get calmer and easier. But experience and time have shown us that life isn't about waiting endlessly for the storm to pass. Life is about being and moving forward even in the rain; and so, I did the same; danced in the rain, with the wind and the storm, until I had practiced patience so much that I became the rainbow after the rain.

This book is a chapter of my life; a reflection of life as seen through Noora's window, that started in despair and gradually became filled by hope, self-love, and deep affection for life.

It is dedicated to you, my dear companion, who so beautifully nurtures the light within you.

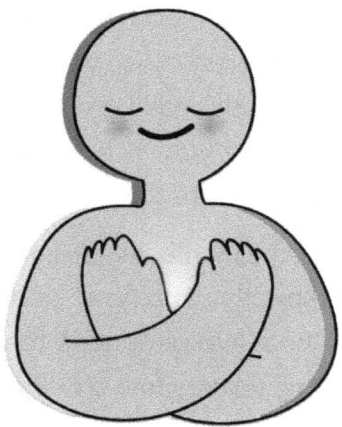

**But Where Did the Story Begin?**
With flowers, gardens, and a budding life with a Noora who was working out, full of passion...
That's truly how it started. It was the beautiful days near spring in Iran, and I was in Vancouver, in the lovely month of February, moving forward on the fast-paced rhythm of life, feeling lost and bewildered. I had a good home, bright with sunlight and moonlight, near Sunset Beach and Starbucks. My job paid well, but I wasn't happy with it. To be honest, I was turning into someone just waiting for the hours to pass so I could escape a foreign land, run, hug the trees in an attempt to blur the exhaustion and homesickness. I remember most nights, I would cry myself to sleep, and now, looking back, I find it striking how deeply I had drowned in that toxic routine, so much so that I didn't even realize crying had become part of my

daily life. But how close was this routine, this life, to the one I had envisioned, planned for, and worked toward? Looking closer, Not only was I no closer to that dream but speeding in an unwanted direction, and that sting was unbearable, and that was not okay.

Still, I won't forget that *despite living in confusion, I experienced countless blessings every day.* Long periods of solitude led me to deepen my friendship with myself, my soul, and my body. It was through this growing self-connection and my body's innate intelligence that I was able to change the course of the game in what happened next.

**From a Small Pain to a Great Awakening**

I was completing stretches following a Saturday morning run, surrounded by fresh air in the heart of Vancouver when all of a sudden I felt a sharp pain stabbing my right breast. The pain kept returning over the following days and weeks until it finally led me to an urgent care clinic.

The doctor there asked a few general questions "Do you drink alcohol? Do you smoke?" then listened to my breathing, checked my heart, and did a quick physical examination. Finally, he told me, "This pain is nothing to worry about. That small, painful lump in your breast is just part of normal breast tissue don't be so sensitive. Go home."

But I trusted my body's intelligence more than his diagnosis. A deep feeling inside told me this couldn't be right. I insisted that he examine me more thoroughly or refer me for a mammogram and further tests. At first, he kept saying it was nothing, but after my persistent requests, he finally gave me the name of another doctor.

That's how, two weeks after that first visit, I found myself lying on an ultrasound bed at a hospital in North Vancouver. In a cold, dimly lit room, a kind female doctor with a soft voice asked me questions "How old are you? What's your lifestyle like?" while taking images of the painful spot in my breast.

After a while, she looked at me and said, "Well, it seems like there's something here." She then scanned under my armpit as well and told me she wanted to get a second opinion from her colleague. She left the room, leaving me alone with my swirling thoughts in that unwelcoming space.

Lying on that cold bed, wrapped in a blanket that barely made a difference, I stared at the monitor. A grid of 32 images was displayed, along with numbers and measurements that made less and less sense the longer I looked at them. As I was still trying to make sense of it all, two female doctors walked back in and started analyzing the images. I understood most of their conversation except for a few unfamiliar medical terms. But one thing was clear: they both agreed that a biopsy was necessary.

I had no idea what a biopsy was, nor had I even heard the word before. I asked the doctor to spell it for me, quickly Googled it, and read: *"A needle biopsy is used to collect tissue samples from suspicious lumps, which are then sent to pathology for analysis."* I even saw some images of bone biopsies, which terrified me. I had no clue how intense my biopsy would be, so I nervously asked the doctor, "Will it hurt?"

She reassured me, "Luckily, it's not from your bone, and the pain is manageable."

Half-joking, I asked, "Manageable for whom?" We both laughed. Laughter was all too brief as she emphasized the serious of her concerns and said: "Noora, whatever it is, we need to do this biopsy. These tiny lumps seem to be spreading, and we need to figure out what they are as soon as possible. If treatment or surgery is necessary, we should act quickly."

The firmness of her tone convinced me to go ahead with the biopsy as a matter of immediacy. I got up from the bed and was soon lying on another, this time in a smaller surgical room, but with better lighting. Two nurses walked in, greeted me warmly, and helped me change into a hospital gown. They sterilized my right breast as to prepare me for my first surgery. The cold sensation of evaporating alcohol on my skin was unsettling. My body felt frozen, and my breathing grew shallow. I pulled my mask down and took a deep breath.

At that moment, an unfamiliar doctor entered the room. He was a tall, broad-shouldered middle-aged man with piercing blue eyes and a gentle voice. "Hello, Noora. How are you, dear? I'm Michael, and I'll be performing your biopsy. How old are you?"

I was stunned, my body tense, my mind racing with wild thoughts. I wanted to crack a joke, maybe ask, *how old do I look?* But I held back, took a breath, and simply smiled.

"Thirty-five," I answered.

He looked surprised. "Really? You look much younger."

I laughed and said, "Yep, and that's my daily challenge having to pull out my ID all the time because no one believes I'm 35. And, on top of that, no one believes I'm Iranian either! People always say I have a European face and Latin energy."

He burst into laughter. "That's an interesting mix!" Then, with a reassuring smile, he added, "I have to say, Noora, your energy is amazing. Let's get this biopsy done quickly. Are you ready?"

In a raspy, movie-style voice, I said, "I WAS BORN READY," and he laughed again, raising his hand for a high-five. His hands were big and warm, carrying a fatherly energy. "Let's get started," he said. I nodded in agreement. But I had no idea that this high energy and lightheartedness would soon turn into tears of pain and deep sighs.

I'm thinking to myself maybe I should explain that this is my way of connecting with people, my defense mechanism to protect my emotions: joking and laughing it off. You'll see more of this as we go.

The biopsy procedure was supervised by a team of three nurses and doctor Micheal. Just as I had suspected, it was essentially a surgery without anesthesia. Painful, bloody, and longer than expected. The first sample was easier to collect than the ones that followed.

When he was taking a sample from under my arm, I experienced a strange kind of pain like someone was stabbing the center of my veins and nerves with a sharp knife. When the pain dragged on, I finally begged the doctor to stop. The entire time, I had turned my face to the other side, avoiding eye contact. But after this excruciating pain kept repeating, I finally looked at him, held his hand with a pleading gaze, and said, "Doctor, please, I'm begging you, stop."

**The Experience of Feeling Light**

Dr. Michael was flustered. He had initially told me the procedure would take 10 to 15 minutes, but by now, I had been under his hands for nearly 40 minutes with four different biopsy needles inserted into my body.

"Noora, please don't move at all. This spot is very sensitive. I don't want to lose it," he said. I whispered, "Okay," as tears streamed down my face.

I wished one of the nurses had been there to hold my hand. The loneliness, combined with the pain, made the moment even harder. I had no choice but to say "okay" and clench my left fist.

And then, suddenly a warm, invisible energy pulled my attention away from pain. For a few seconds, I felt as if God was right beside my bed. More than ever before, I could feel His presence.

I clenched my fist tighter, took a deep breath, and closed my eyes. Strangely, no image remained in my mind just the pure sensation of His presence.

With all its ups and downs, the biopsy was finally completed. Dr. Michael, his hands slightly bloodstained, bid me farewell. Two nurses came to bandage the biopsy site. One of them, helped me sit up and said, "I know that was a huge challenge for you. How much pain are you in? Do you want some juice or cookies?"

My eyes were still filled with tears. "A lot. Can you hold my hand?" I deeply wished she would hug me, but I didn't say it.

They bandaged my upper body, put fresh surgical tape on me, and gave me a new gown. "Head to the mammography room," they instructed.

## A Step Further

I could no longer walk normally, bent slightly to my right, hugging myself, following the shooting pain, my focus was disrupted, laboring the process of even finding the mammography room. I heard someone calling my name, thankfully it was the mammography technician, and I was able to correct my course.

She was a woman with incredible positive energy. When she saw me wincing in pain, she approached me warmly. "Hi, Noora. I'm Dr. Jacqueline, and we'll be taking images of your breast today."

Noticing my distress, she comforted me, saying, "Noora, I know how much courage it takes to go through all of this in one day. I'm proud of you. No matter what the results say, I know you'll get through it."

She looked straight into my eyes as she said it.

I was exhausted and overwhelmed. I thanked her, wishing so badly I could hug her, but I didn't.

After a bloody and painful introduction to medical tests, it was relieving to discover mammography took a less invasive approach. No needles, no radioactive substances, no blood tests just a little pressure, which was bearable.

As she took the necessary images, she attempted to

make me laugh which reminded me of myself and helped raise the levity of the situation.

After 30 minutes, we were done. I thanked her and said, "Thank you for being so full of kindness and expressing it. I hope I never see you here again."

She let out a big laugh and replied, "You're full of energy yourself, and I'm sure whatever happens, you'll handle it."

We said our goodbyes. I closed the door behind me and walked away.

"What a Day..."

In just three hours, I had gone from a healthy young woman to a young woman who had major medical tests. I was exhausted. I was overwhelmed; I was scared. I left the hospital frightened and sat at a bus stop with an ice pack pressed against a breast, further amplifying the pain. I held onto a packet of painkillers and with tear-filled eyes I sat there, heartbroken, I had endured it all alone.

I was in shock. Stunned. I hadn't been ready for this much to happen in one day.

Even though the doctor and nurses advised me to go home and rest, I couldn't afford to lose that day's wages. So, despite everything, I dragged myself back to work. But if something similar happens to you please listen to your body's needs and follow it. Money comes and goes and remember the most important responsibility is taking care of ourselves not people's businesses. I didn't. I should have been more caring toward myself.

**Light in the Shadow of Uncertainty**

A lot changed over the next 3 weeks, I left my job, got a better one, and started my first month under so much pressure while the pain of the biopsy persisted. In the middle of an important meeting, an unknown number called me. It was a new doctor. She said, "We need to meet. And please bring a close friend with you." I said OKAY, but I had no intention of doing so. I thought to myself, in this day and age, everyone has their worries; I don't want to burden anyone with mine.

So, I took a day off and went straight to the doctor's office. She was a young Indian woman who introduced herself as Taran. She examined me thoroughly and then said, "Please have a seat, Noora." I sat down. She took a deep breath and said, "Alright, Noora, although everything seems normal in this physical examination, and your body appears healthy, the tests you took last week don't bring good news. The biopsy shows that cancer cells in your body are multiplying rapidly. It's an aggressive cancer that has spread to other parts of your body, and you need to start serious treatment as soon as possible."

As she spoke, I saw nothing but fear in her eyes. She was

trying to stay composed, but she stuttered slightly. Despite her demeanor, my mind remained calm. My feelings were reflected in my composed expression, and I immediately began asking, "This type of cancer you can treat, right? It's curable, right? What will the treatment be like?"

She replied, "There are different options. We need to determine which one is best for you," and continued explaining. I was listening, but I wasn't really hearing her. Yet as she spoke, I understood the gravity of the situation on some level. Images from others' lives, primarily family, began flashing before me, and I thought about the things I had left to do, and I was certain this wasn't the end.

She asked, "Noora, are you okay? Do you want me to call a friend to come pick you up? You shouldn't be alone right now."

I said, "No, thank you. Can I get a copy of my test results?"

"Of course, of course," she said and left me in a daze to make the copies.

At that moment, I thought about how much this doctor's office felt like a prison, cold and uninviting. If I were in their place, I would give such news in a bright, comforting room. I believe space has an incredible impact, and regardless of the severity of the diagnosis, I would talk about treatment in a way that felt more hopeful. But maybe my opinion was the least important thing at that moment.

A nursing student had been in the room the whole time, taking notes. Her gaze was full of kindness. She said, "Noora, you're so young. I hope your healthy lifestyle helps you recover quickly."

I smiled and said, "I'm sure it will."

I wanted to hug her, I needed to feel a connection with another person, and reduce the panic inherent throughout this situation but at this moment, I restrained myself, knowing they were professionals and couldn't give me support in every area.

The sun was shining beautifully on the street outside. The clinic was very close to my house, just a five-minute walk. Sunlight and moonlight were both within my reach.

When I got home, I felt lost. I was too "okay" for someone with an advanced, aggressive disease. My family's faces kept flashing before my eyes. I sat on my couch, and suddenly, the tears started flowing. For a few moments, my entire journey up to that point played before my eyes.

I didn't want to overthink it.

I got up, turned on my laptop and speakers, played some music, and danced while the tears kept falling.

(God only knows what I was feeling and what was about to come.)

### A Little Before This...

Sometimes I think about how, since September 2022, when I arrived in Canada on a student visa, I never really felt anything different about this place. I had traveled a lot before, and I had come to believe that no matter where I was, life would support me.

During my first two years in this new country, while I was living in the beautiful city of Vancouver, a revolution had broken out in Iran. The distance from home and witnessing my people's pain tore at my already exhausted spirit. As always, my defense mechanism was to keep myself busy, I filled my life with multiple jobs, pushing forward (or maybe backward, who knows?).

For a year, I lived in a dorm while studying and working three jobs. One of them I loved, another I tolerated, and I had also found a volunteer role that I adored. In the gaps between all this, I studied intensely and became one of my professors' favorite students.

For the job I barely tolerated, I had to wake up at 4 AM, finish work before 7 AM, have breakfast, and then head to my second job, which I loved social media marketing for a fast-food restaurant until 4 PM. After that, I'd run to the library, do my assignments, attend classes from 6 to 9 PM, and if I had any energy left, I'd go to the gym. I exhausted myself so much that by the time I got home, I could only think about deep sleep.

Three days a week, I volunteered for the position I was truly passionate about, helping international students. My hard work and positive energy helped me settle into university life much faster than expected. From the beginning, I had started guiding other students, sharing my experiences, helping them find jobs, and introducing them to university services that could make their lives easier. Passion for service radiated from me, and everyone around me could see that Noora loved to help.

That passion worked wonders. The university soon offered me a part-time job, which I accepted. At the start of 2023, I moved into my new office at the heart of TWU's beautiful Langley campus, ready to shine even more.

Like many Canadian universities, ours had students from countless nationalities. I loved engaging with such diverse cultures, helping, and contributing value. I knew exactly what I was meant to do and how I could be useful.

This, along with my love for life and joy, led me to organize beautiful, high-quality cultural events, all voluntarily. Everyone was amazed at how much I did. No matter how busy I was, I always made time for all kinds of volunteer works.

At these events, I invited everyone from the university president to the chaplain and faculty members. These programs, which introduced different cultures, were new experiences for them too, so they attended eagerly, enjoyed themselves and our friendships deepened.

With this whirlwind of busyness, I got through my first year embracing every hardship at my beloved Trinity Western University.

Sometimes, I think I kept myself so busy to escape the shadow of a great sorrow that sometimes loomed over my life. But after all that, graduating and getting a work permit, I finally started to feel a sense of stability in my life. I had moved to downtown Vancouver. Amid all this outward success, I never could have imagined, not even in my dreams, that I would soon be facing advanced breast cancer.

**Back to the Present...**

After my doctor's appointment all my doctor's words having previously gone over my head.... I remembered she had little advice to offer me in dealing with my new situation.

I had no thoughts or images of what was to come. My mind was completely blank.

But one thing was clear: I didn't fully accept how bad my health situation was.

What I did register was that this, too, was just another experience.

I pictured it this way: I was hosting an uninvited guest for an unknown period, one who was here to give me a different kind of life experience.

My focus was on starting serious treatment. But one thing was for sure I didn't want chemotherapy. I didn't want to lose my hair.

After ten years of having short hair, I finally decided to grow it this year so I could braid it and let my mother weave her hands through it when I saw her for Nowruz in 2025.

That was my plan.

But clearly, life had a different one.

What choice did I have?

Nothing.

Just keep going.

Now, a year later, looking back, I realize that despite the overwhelming fear, I made great progress in my health situation. Felt like I jumped from a height so great that I couldn't see the ground, yet I closed my eyes, my legs shaking, and jumped.

Somehow, I knew this wouldn't last forever. And that, eventually, my wings would open, and I would see the Earth and its beauties again.

**The Courage to Live in the Shadows**

Yesterday, I had my first phone conversation with my oncology specialist. By the end of our discussion, I made a firm decision to start chemotherapy. Uncertain and unaware of what lay ahead, I put my trust in the supportive force of life and embarked on my treatment journey. Looking back, I believe this was the moment my faith came to my aid. From the very beginning, I embraced my physical, emotional, and spiritual well-being, reassuring myself that, by God's grace, I would receive everything I needed to heal. I was certain that my body and soul would follow suit.

However, this was only half the truth as alongside such positive thoughts, a flood of negative ones also surged. Thoughts like, "Why me? How could this happen when I've lived such a healthy and mindful life?" Yet I managed to catch myself as these thoughts arose. No! Not even for a second could I let myself be trapped in that mindset. Those thoughts would only drag me down into despair, into the role of a victim something I refused to become.

It's easy to justify feeling unlucky, lonely, and miserable. It's easy to believe no one sees you, to think that if you were to disappear in this lonely room, no one would hear you cry. That all your efforts would be in vain. That life is unfair, cruel, and meaningless. But I realized something, life has never been fair. Maybe, just maybe, my role is to make the world a place where people can feel a little more secure and a little more just. As my beloved Gandhi said, I must be the change I wish to see in the world.

Logically speaking, it didn't make sense for me to be my own worst enemy. Why should I drain my own strength when I needed every ounce of it? I knew what I wanted. And this difficult experience taught me how to extract the best possible outcome from it. When I saw that the train of negative thoughts was taking me nowhere, I got off. I paused. I reflected.

I stood at the crossroads between fading hope and deep despair. This choice was akin to an internal battle, one that needed to be fought over and over, even moment by moment. I had to stay alert, making sure I didn't get on the wrong train. The unpredictable nature of my situation only made it clearer this time, the choice was real. This was no game.

With immense effort, I had to sift through countless thoughts and carefully select the ones that would propel me forward. Thankfully, I was already somewhat used to this process. When I look at the decisions I've made throughout my life, I see that I've been a good gardener, carefully tending to my growth. I've taken responsibility, nurtured my potential, and stood by myself through thick and thin.

I've made many good decisions. And, of course, as a human being, I've also made my share of mistakes some of them painful. There were times when, overwhelmed by suffering, I wanted to throw everything away. I wanted to shake my fist at the universe and demand an explanation why did I have to endure so much pain just to learn a lesson?

But after all the tears and frustration, I would find myself on my knees, in deep silence. Completely surrendered. Still.

I think we've all been there wrestling with life's challenges, struggling to make sense of it all. But after everything, the greatest lesson I've learned is this: even when I thought I had everything under control, life had its way of reminding me otherwise. The real question became, now that this has happened, how can I move forward? What's the best thing to do to make this situation better?

Overwhelmed by the sheer weight of everything, I took refuge in silence. I had no energy to analyze, question, or resist anymore. And now, looking back, I see that was the right thing to do. Sometimes, the best response is to slow down, let go of entitlement, and simply pause to listen. In my case, stillness and surrender illuminated the path ahead.

In the deepest layers of my being, I built a sanctuary a place of peace and resilience. I emerged from my confusion, stronger in my faith and patience, and then, I turned my attention to whatever I could do to make things better, no matter what had already happened.

**May 6, 2024 – My Home, Heart of Vancouver**

Lately, I've had a lot of phone calls for my upcoming appointments, check-ups, and medication schedules. Every time I see an unknown number on my phone, I feel a wave of anxiety. It's as if my body has become a reservoir of hidden stress, now being forced to the surface. All the fears and worries I had unknowingly buried for years seem to be unraveling now.

It appears to me that some version of this happens frequently to most people. I want you to really reflect on this. Be mindful. And after reading this book, promise me you won't fall into the same traps again.

I promise you this it's never too late to start taking care of yourself. No matter how hard things get, there's always something to be grateful for. Ahkhkh I didn't like to say this cliche but based on life experiences, things could always be worse. At least now I know that if I start treatment, I'll have more than five months to live. Whatever happened in the past is behind me. The most important thing is that I am now living a more aware version of myself. In this new phase, my commitment is to preserve this gift of awareness as much as possible.

**My dear body, I love you now more than ever.**

At one of my medical appointments, I was scheduled to meet a surgeon to assess whether I needed surgery. It was at a new hospital, in a cold examination room, while "what ifs" raced through my mind. I put on the hospital gown and waited. After fifteen minutes, she arrived. A slightly older woman with large gray eyes, thick glasses, and a mask covering her face.

I had Googled her name beforehand and found out she was one of Canada's top surgeons an esteemed professor who had authored multiple books and research papers on breast cancer, and a renowned expert in her field.

She asked me to lie down and began asking me various questions about my symptoms and physical changes. After examining me, she said, "Well, Noora, everything looks good. Despite the advanced nature of your illness, fortunately, you don't need surgery now. We have excellent medications for your treatment, and we hope they'll work well for you."

My eyes widened with excitement. Her words filled me with the most comforting relief. Surgery and losing a part of my body had been my biggest fears. Even though I had tried not to think about it, I felt a huge weight had been lifted off my shoulders. Overcome with emotion, my eyes filled with tears. I thanked her, wanting to hug her but I didn't. Instead, I left.

On my way home, I kept my hand over my breast, whispering words of gratitude. This beautiful part of my body would stay with me, and together, we would celebrate full recovery.

Lately, I've developed a new and beautiful habit of talking to my body more often. Every time I step into the shower, I sing, "I am blessed and healed." The only things I listen to on YouTube are guided meditations for complete health. I breathe deeper. I let the sunlight warm my skin. I give thanks for every sip of water, and every bite of food, knowing that they are cleansing my body of illness.

As I increasingly acknowledged how thankful I was for seemingly forgotten elements of everyday life, I began to believe that miracles are unfolding in things we take for granted.

And you, my dear girl Noora!

I must tell you how much I love this about you, the way even in the darkest moments, you remain patient and faithful, always searching for light. You continue to celebrate life, reminding those around you to do the same.

I won't lie and say I was never afraid. Even now, a year into my treatment, every small pain in my breast terrifies me. But alongside fear, I also feel my deep love for life the force that gives me the strength to move forward.

And through it all, I know one thing for sure: He sees me. He knows my heart. And He is the one guiding my way.

**Spreading the News**

With all my strength, I was trying to manage my emotions. It went well for a while, but I still hadn't gathered the courage to openly face the reality of my Stage 4 breast cancer, with metastasis to the lymph nodes under my left armpit and clavicle. I certainly didn't share this with my family first, but oddly enough, the first person I felt comfortable telling was my financial advisor. He immediately sprang into action, trying to figure out if there was any way to get financial support from my active insurance policies so I could go through treatment with some peace of mind. Chemotherapy had physically drained me so much that I had to quit my job, I was relying on updates from him daily. At the end, not even a single cent came through.

The second person who needed to know was my boss. Ramadan was approaching, so I told her the situation and asked her not to forget me in her prayers. But her reaction was strange. When she realized how serious and intense my treatment would be, she became visibly upset, and I could see a wave of hopelessness and pity in her eyes which I absolutely hated. I told her, "I thought people of strong faith should show more hope and resilience in difficult times."

She replied, "Noora, you're young, athletic, and full of energy. It's such a shame for you to be taken away."

I wanted to laugh out of sheer frustration. I was sure no one could have handled this conversation worse than she just did. I tried to compose myself and said, "I understand that you're upset." Then, I reminded her of a verse from the Quran that she was memorizing daily: La taqnatu min rahmatillah. "Do not despair of the mercy of Allah."

Seeing that sickening look of pity in her eyes made me feel even worse. I couldn't stand it any longer, so I quickly said goodbye.

I rushed to the restroom, splashed cold water on my face, and tried to shake off the drained feeling that short conversation had left me with. I forced myself to forget her sorrowful expression. Instead, I used my "stare-at-yourself" technique I looked straight into my own honey-colored eyes in the mirror. They stared back at me, full of hope, and I felt a deep love for myself. Oh God, how much I loved these moments of meeting myself. How sweet they were! My heart felt warm and alive, and I said out loud, "I am choosing to hold onto this warmth and love for life."

Then, with a smile, I added, "Noora, you do realize how madly in love I am with you, right?"

I swore to myself that I would always take the best care of myself. "Pull yourself together, girl. We've got a lot to do."

I felt significantly better. As I stepped out of the restroom, a cool breeze hit my damp face. I shivered but felt refreshed. I smiled, took a deep breath, and went off to tell the next important person.

That next person was someone special. After a decade of being single, I finally decided to enter a meaningful and beautiful relationship. I had been seeing him for exactly two weeks. A self-made, charming Canadian man. He knew I was getting various medical tests done, but he assumed they were just routine checkups. And now, he was about to be the third person to know what was going on.

As hard as it was, I had to tell him. He needed to decide if he wanted to stay and go through this with me or if he'd rather say, "It was nice knowing you, take care," and walk away.

I had no idea how he'd react. So, I texted him:

Me: "Hey, how's your day going? I want to see you; we need to talk." Him: "Heeey Noora! Seeing your message made me happy. I was just about to text you myself. How about 4:45 today?"

We met up. After about ten minutes of chatting and laughing, I looked into his eyes and said, "Jordan, remember how you always joked about how organized I am with my doctor checkups? And how you told me you haven't been to a doctor since you were 12? We laughed so much about that."

He chuckled. "I swear I wasn't lying." We laughed briefly, then he said, "So...?"

After a few seconds of silence, I told him, "I'm sorry, I hate saying this, but all those tests show that there's a very small tumor in my breast, and it's spreading fast. I need to start serious treatment soon."

I explained to him how this would change me: I would lose my hair, I would become weak, and I might lose my ability to have children due to the side effects of the medication. There would be days when I'd feel drained, and maybe even more changes that I couldn't predict. However, my doctors were very hopeful because of my age and physical strength.

He listened intently the entire time, staring at me with a

mixture of focus and disbelief.

I asked him, "Tell me what you're thinking. How do you feel?"

His eyes were full of unspoken questions, but he simply said, "Let's start your treatment. Of course, all the hardship is on you, but Noora, I don't know anything about this. I need you to teach me, tell me what I need to do and when. Okay?"

I nodded. "Okay."

This was new for both of us but knowing that we were both focused on finding a solution gave me comfort. Neither of us had experience with this. We didn't know what was coming. But he looked at me with his honey-brown eyes, his soft, pinkish face, and said, "Noora, I don't want this to be the reason we part ways."

I asked, "Are you sure?"

He said, "Of course, I'm sure."

But I still had doubts. I didn't want his response to be driven by emotions or pity. Then suddenly, I snapped out of my overthinking mode I shut down my analytical brain, leaned in, and hugged him. A hug to make up for all the ones I had wanted to give but hadn't.

Now, as I write this, it has been about two months since my last chemotherapy dose, and, for some reasons, I will explain later, he is no longer a part of Noora's new life.

But I have to say, his presence during the toughest moments was truly valuable. Despite our cultural and linguistic differences, our journey aligned in many ways and sometimes diverged. Like every relationship sometimes sunny, sometimes foggy. But there was always respect between us, and in the end, we parted with that same respect.

Phew. That was hard; really hard. But the past is the past. Now, let's talk about what happened next.

**May 10, 2024 – Vancouver**

Hello from a beautiful sunny day

It's Tuesday. Two weeks have passed since my last doctor's appointment. One of my medical tests, the PET scan, confirmed what my doctors had suspected—the cancer was spreading and had reached another spot, right under my clavicle, close to my carotid artery. They need to take a biopsy from that area.

I looked at my doctor in despair and said, "The last biopsy was really painful."

He replied, "I know, Noora. But I'm worried, and I need to be sure what this mass under your clavicle is so we can adjust your treatment dosage. Please endure it and get it done."

I had already committed to trusting the process, so I told myself once again: Be aware that at the beginning of this journey, you will have to hear, see, and process things you never wanted to. But you must go through it hand in hand with your medical team.

For the thousandth time, I was scared. And for the thousand-and-first time, I said, "Okay. It seems I have no choice but to trust this process."

So, the plan was set for tomorrow, I'd have a clavicle biopsy and three new blood tests. And then, at exactly 1:30 p.m. on Thursday, I would receive my first dose of chemotherapy. The road ahead was unknown. But I was determined to walk it.

**In the Shadow of Fearful Awareness**

With an fervent obsession, I collect every medical report from doctors and nurses. I've asked them the name and type of my illness a hundred times, and a hundred times I've forgotten. So, I dug through these reports to find the exact name of my cancer. During this time, I started watching countless YouTube videos of people who had faced similar challenges and overcome them.

I promised myself that even if I couldn't find an inspiring

video, I would roll up my sleeves and be the first to create one. Since I didn't find much engaging Persian content, I decided to make my own. After some time passed in my chemotherapy journey, I shared my videos on YouTube and Instagram.

From time to time, I came across terrifying links about chemotherapy side effects and how to prepare for them. Alas, they were of no use to me and even became damaging, so I deleted all those links from my Google history. I strongly recommend that you don't seek out content that drains your courage especially if, like me, you're alone and have a powerful imagination. You know that imagination can be your greatest blessing or, in an instant, knock you to the ground.

## The Biopsy of My Cancerous Mass and the Biopsy of My Faith

On the day of my second biopsy, I went to my usual hospital. A very thin, young nurse with Asian features handed me a fresh gown to wear.

Despite this being my second biopsy, my mind, thoughts, and fears still accompanied me. I lay on the bed as a very young-looking doctor approached. She appeared to be Iranian, wearing a brown floral outfit, with golden-highlighted hair and jewelry that shimmered around her ears and neck. It seemed she would be the one performing my biopsy.

She stood over me and said, "Hello, Noora. I'm Dr. Malahat. How are you? How old are you?"

I replied, "Hello, Dr. Malahat. I'm good and thank you for asking. Honestly, I'm a little stressed. I'm 35 years old. May I ask, are you Iranian?"

She said, "Yes, I am."

I responded, "That's so cool! I'm Iranian too!"

She raised an eyebrow and said, "Really? You don't look Iranian at all."

Inside, I groaned, Oh God, not this question again! But outwardly, I smiled and enthusiastically replied, "But you look very Iranian!" My excitement was obvious.

I explained my comment further: "Iranian people take great care of themselves, just like Koreans."

Our entire conversation was in English. She let out a brief, unamused laugh. It was clear she didn't appreciate my comment. Her face turned serious.

She said, "Noora, the area where we need to take the biopsy is very sensitive. We might hit your carotid artery, which could cause bleeding. But don't worry, we'll take care of you."

All the excitement and reassurance I had felt vanished,

replaced by fear and doubt.

As I looked into her eyes, I saw a particular uncertainty. I asked her, "Is there any other way to do the biopsy?"

She said, "No. This is the only way. But don't worry!"

That phrase, don't worry, had never made me this worried before. It was completely ineffective.

I felt like crying, but I didn't.

At that moment, a group of medical students entered the room to observe and learn from my biopsy. They all greeted me, and I waved back at them.

This was serious. There was no escaping it. But what if she hit my artery?

I had to stop these thoughts. Well, I had no other choice.

So, I turned to my magic wand, faith. Instead of dwelling on my fears, I chose to trust the doctor's words.

I collected myself, clasped my hands together, closed my eyes to the doctors in the room, and opened them to my heart. I began speaking to God:

> *"God, I know these people are here to help me. Thank you for giving them the skill and ability to do this perfectly, without pain or bleeding. Everything will go smoothly."*

I took a deep breath and whispered, "Thank you, thank

you."

Dr. Malahat asked, "Noora, are you okay? We're about to start."

I opened my eyes, looked into hers, and said, "I trust in your expertise."

She gave me a small smile and began the procedure.

After 15 minutes of various attempts, the biopsy was completed from beneath my carotid artery without a single drop of blood or an ounce of pain.

Dr. Malahat thanked me for my confidence and cooperation. Truthfully, I was grateful to her too. I felt a deep sense of pride. I knew, once again, that my unwavering faith had been rewarded.

I gave myself a big, tight hug. I was proud of my trust, my courage, and my ever-faithful companion God.

## Next Steps...

My next appointment with my oncologist is in two weeks. Dr. Bernard is a young, serious, and highly skilled Canadian doctor. This will be my second time seeing him. He is my primary doctor, and we meet once every three weeks before I receive my medication. Each time before our appointment, I must take a blood test so he can check whether my blood health is stable enough for chemotherapy.

During our first meeting, he gave me my treatment plan. According to it, I need to receive at least eight doses of chemotherapy, meaning my schedule for the next eight months is set. However, he also told me that changes might be made to this plan, things could be added or removed.

Along with the treatment plan, they provided me with a lot of additional information, especially about the side effects of my medications. Reading through them, I wasn't sure if I'd be able to handle it all. But the document also stated: "These side effects may occur, but not necessarily." Dr. Bernard is very logical. He suggested that I reach out to a wig bank to get a synthetic wig or a head covering. He also handed me a list of medications to take before chemotherapy to help control severe nausea.

Then he asked, "Were you able to get a visa for your family members to come?" I had no answer. With deep disappointment, I replied, "Not yet… I haven't even told them I'm going through this."

He looked at me in surprise and said, "You need to talk to them." I answered, "I just can't right now. I don't have the strength."

I took the papers from him, feeling overwhelmed and restless. I longed for my mom, my sisters, my dad, my brother, my sister-in-law, my brothers-in-law, my nieces and nephews, longed for all the hugs in the world. Yet, after all these days and unexpected news, I still hadn't found the courage to face myself in the mirror, let alone my family. The loneliness was suffocating me.

Writing these words is like reliving my pain, bringing tears to my eyes and aches my heart. But I promised myself that my story would be honest. I want to shed light on the things that are often left unspoken, the feelings we all might experience in similar or even different situations. There are steep uphill battles and sharp downhill slides, and sometimes, we reach peaceful valleys. Through it all, we are alive in our emotions, filled with fear and hope, light and darkness. And I, the main character of this journey, know that my beliefs shape my path, and my actions determine the outcome.

## The First Day of Chemotherapy

I woke up early. The sunrise painted the sky in warm hues, ready to shine with all its might. I loved it. As I laced up my running shoes, I softly sang to myself: "The sun is shining, filling me with joy."

I went down the stairs and started a slow jog, making my way to nature. I sang different hymns, embraced the trees, and caressed the branches; I love doing that.

You remember, right? My core belief is that life always supports me, and I support life in return. I love this partnership.

When I got home, I took a shower, had a high-protein breakfast, and got ready to go to the hospital. My energy was soaring, I felt like I could fly.

At the hospital, it was crowded. It was a warm day, and the rooms were filled with patients, nurses, and their companions.

They showed me to my bed, which was next to an overweight gay couple with serious, grumpy expressions. They kept murmuring complaints under their breath. My first medication was administered, and suddenly, their loud voices filled the room with the darkest conversation:

"This is just the beginning. You're in for hell." "These nurses will poke you a hundred times before finding a vein."

"The side effects are going to wreck you."

They weren't speaking to me directly, but the room was small, and their voices were loud. Whether I wanted to or not, I heard every word. I glanced at them occasionally. I tried not to listen, but it was impossible. I attempted to lighten the mood by smiling and making small talk about the weather. It wasn't enough.

To prevent their negativity from poisoning my spirit, I asked my nurse to draw the curtain around my chair, both to block them from my view and subtly protest their energy. After all, I was going to be here for at least three hours, and I had filled myself with positivity and light. I couldn't allow myself to be dragged into a toxic space.

For the final medication the one with the worst side effects the nurse suggested I wear ice gloves to protect my fingernails. I had no idea what these gloves looked like, but I thought about keeping my nails healthy and agreed.

They brought them over, and the moment I put them on, I regretted it. Within the first ten minutes, the icy burn seeped into my bones. Tears welled up in my eyes, but my hands were trapped in the heavy, frozen gloves, so I couldn't wipe them away. My nurse noticed and, with a furrowed brow, said, "Noora, I'm so sorry. I know this hurts, but sweetheart, it's necessary to save your nails."

Now, two months after my last chemotherapy session, I see the side effects appearing on my toenails. And I feel so grateful that I endured that pain back then. Otherwise, I would have lost the nails on my hands too, making everything even harder.

**Chemotherapy and Saying Goodbye to My Hair**

After receiving the first dose of chemotherapy, I kept checking my hair every moment, hoping it wouldn't fall out, and God knows how happy I felt when my hair seemed to resist. I even thought to myself, there's no way my hair will fall out. But exactly one week before receiving the second dose, my hair started falling out aggressively. Within two to three days, I lost 70% of my hair, and then with the help of my friend Nadia and her husband Nima, who had dealt with a similar issue, we shaved my head. I had so much hair that their first hair clippers broke, and my friend's husband went out and bought a new one right away to finish cutting my hair.

In the dark tunnel of chemotherapy, every time after receiving the medication, the side effects made me feel like I was at the end of my life. At least, that's how it was for me, especially after the third dose of chemotherapy. But, as I always say: "There is always something to be thankful for," and this time, it was a good reason. Right after the second dose, when I examined my breast, I found that the little invasive lump was no longer there. I was sure that my efforts to care for my words, thoughts, and actions would pay off, so I made another appointment with my dear doctor to discuss it.

**The First Glimmer of Light in the Darkness**

On my way to the doctor's office, I kept my hand on my breast, talking to it and thanking it for healing so quickly. All these inner conversations were multiplying my energy and bringing a big smile to my face. When I reached the reception, two young women, greeted me, and I told them, "What a beautiful day! I have an appointment with Dr. Bernard." They asked me to sit down, and a nurse called my name to take my weight.

I stepped on the scale, and it showed that I had lost about two kilograms in three weeks, and everything seemed normal. While waiting to see my doctor, I felt like this moment was important and impactful, so I took out my phone and took some pictures and videos. Just then, I heard Dr. Bernard's voice saying, "Hello Noora, it's good to see you. Let's see what's going on today!" I laughed out loud and said, "I'm sure it's good news," and we walked into his office, the same small and cold room.

Dr. Bernard quickly pulled up my file on his system and began reading all the tests and reports from other doctors. I watched his face carefully, paying attention to his small gray eyes. By the way, I don't think I've told you this, but I am strangely fascinated by watching people's faces, and this time, alongside this observation, I expected positive reactions from Dr. Bernard's body language and face. It was satisfying to see my suspicions confirmed as he gave a brief smile. Seeing that smile on his serious face was like seeing a shooting star in the night sky for me. He looked at me and started asking various questions: "How have you felt about the treatment so far? What bothered you? What did you do to address it?" I answered his questions patiently, and he asked if I had any questions. I replied, "Doctor, I want to make sure about something with your help." He said, "Of course, what is it?"

I asked him to examine my breast to make sure that I wasn't imagining things and that the little lump was truly gone. He agreed, "Sure, let's do it." He examined me, moving his fingers gently around the lymph nodes under my arms and neck. He closed his eyes to be more precise in his work. He checked my throat, neck, and ear, and said, "Yes, you're right. I also feel that the little invasive lump is no longer there. But it's a bit strange that it's gone after just two doses. I need to sent you in for another another scan to make sure everything is clear!"

A beautiful sense of excitement replaced any doubt in my heart, and I squeezed my hands tightly together to thank my body at that moment. Dr. Bernard was a thoughtful person who always spoke based on the latest research, studies, and tests. He said, "Noora, I have to tell you that we are happy and surprised because your treatment seems to be progressing very well, and our newest medications are working great for you. Your blood quality is excellent, and we're happy that, considering how heavy the treatment was, you're handling it so well," he said whilst keeping his statuesque expression fixed. I focused intensely, watching his facial expressions, hearing these words, and enjoying every moment. I was proud of myself; it was so sweet to see that the things I had been doing with my heart to heal myself were both logical and effective according to science.

Dr. Bernard also said, "Noora, keep doing whatever you're doing whether it's exercise, meditation, dietary changes, or anything else." He helped me sit down, and tears of joy and gratitude filled my eyes. I thanked him a lot. He said, "I'll see you in three weeks. Take care of yourself," and he said goodbye. I was left with so many good feelings, and that room was no longer cold or small.

Two weeks later, I went for my new PET scan at the hospital. During those two weeks, I kept declaring myself blessed and healed. Whether in the shower, before bed, during exercise, eating, drinking, or every time I looked at myself in the mirror. My scan was late in the day, and by the time I reached the hospital, I was very hungry and tired. Just for your information, if you're going for a PET scan, it's usually in the afternoon because you must fast for at least six hours before and can only drink water. I had followed these instructions.

At the reception, some pleasant music was playing on the radio, and I started gently swaying to it, shaking out the stress from my body. I handed over my treatment card and filled out the necessary forms, waiting while carefully observing everything. The last time, I had been completely absorbed in my thoughts, but this time, even the plain blue color of the waiting room chairs seemed interesting and noticeable. Just then, the scan technician called my name, "Noora?"

It was the same Korean guy who had done my scan last time. I was happy to see him; he had this calm, reassuring energy with a beautiful smile on his face that eased my stress. This time, I stood up cheerfully and said, "I'm here," and greeted him in Korean. He smiled and said, "How are you?" I answered, "Gamsahabnida, good," half Korean, half English and we both laughed at my creative mix.

I told him, "I have some fresh news for you," then lowered my voice and said, "Kim, I'm sure my illness is gone now, and I came today to gather evidence with the pictures you'll take to prove my claim." He looked at me with excited eyes and said, "Oh! Really? I hope that's the case."

He guided me to the room where the radioactive substance was going to be injected. He checked my blood pressure and blood sugar; my sugar was normal, and my blood pressure was 5.5, which proved that fasting had had an effect. Then they started the IV and pump, and whilst he worked and guided me through these procedures the joy and optimism I'd felt at the beginning didn't wane. He was a professional, and his voice had a kind, masculine tone. The last time I told him about my love for K-pop and BTS, and how I knew enough Korean to greet people. He got excited. When it was time to take the IV, I sat in the special chair. He asked, "Are you ready, Nona?"

With a big smile, I said, "Noora, not Nona." He replied, "Then your studies haven't reached this part yet," and we laughed. I realized that in Korean culture, "Nona" is a respectful way of addressing women, especially when you're unsure if they're older or younger. I said, "Aha, that's cool! So, from now on, I'm Nona Noora." We both laughed, and he said, "Nona Noora, take a deep breath," and very smoothly and perfectly found the vein, connected the IV, and injected the radioactive material. Afterward, he put a warm blanket on me, dimmed the lights so I could rest, and left me alone for 45 minutes.

Again, I was left in that small, dark room, with just myself and the thoughts swirling in my head. I was so tired. I tried to sleep, but I couldn't. I grabbed my phone, played a YouTube worship, and repeatedly imagined myself healed, blessed, and eager to serve life. Maybe I dozed off a bit, but I was jolted awake by the sound of a knock. "How was your rest, Noora?" He asked. I said, "Good, but I really want to sleep well." He replied, "I know you're tired, but we need to go for the scan," and helped me get up. I was a bit dizzy, so he held my hand and said, "You had a tough day, but it'll be over soon." I pulled myself together and said, "Yeah, let's go."

We headed toward the room where the PET scan tunnel was. It was a tunnel with more patterns and less noise than the MRI tunnel. Overall, I prefer the PET scan to the MRI, except for the injection part. I was in the machine for about 20 minutes, keeping my thoughts positive as they wildly wandered everywhere. I thought about the beautiful motivations in my life, the trip I would take to Iran immediately after completing my treatment, and the afternoon Cardamom tea with my parents. During these thoughts, the scan was completed.

My Korean friend said the results would be sent to my doctor within 48 hours. I asked, "What do you think?" He said, "Noora, we're not allowed to comment, but I hope everything goes well." I replied, "Gamzahamida," which means "Thank you," and he smiled and said, "Take care of yourself." I said, "You too," and we wished each other goodnight. He guided me to the exit. It was 8 PM, and we were almost the last people in the hospital. The automatic doors opened and closed, and I took a taxi back home.

A week later, my next appointment was with Dr. Bernard, but he wasn't there. He had gone on a conference trip, and a colleague saw me. Her name was very hard to remember, but she told me that Dr. Bernard really wanted to give me the news himself. However, he had to attend this conference, where they would discuss my case and present my treatment results to many specialists. My new doctor was very pleased with my test results, which were visible on her monitor, and said, "Noora, everything is progressing better than we planned. Congratulations!" I extended my hand for a handshake and said, "I knew it, I was sure of it. Thank you very much." She said, "This PET scan also confirms that the disease is not present in your body, but this type of cancer is aggressive, and if it's not fully treated, there's a risk of relapse. We'll need to continue chemotherapy for five more doses to be sure the treatment is complete."

When I thought about the side effects of chemotherapy, I didn't want to agree, but I had already decided to fully recover I needed to listen to my healthcare team.

So, I said, "I'm ready. We'll do whatever you recommend, even though it's hard, and it's even harder alone."

Doctor said, "We'll give you a letter so you can bring your family members to be with you." I thanked her. She immediately wrote the letter and handed it to me. I later placed it with the rest of the documents for my sister to bring them to me, but our tourist visa application was rejected in less than 48 hours.

Let's return to my conversation with the doctor, who insisted that I shouldn't consider my treatment finished and should continue with chemotherapy. I listened and committed myself to the process.

Don't you think that hearing this good news would make enduring the next doses easier?

Of course, it would!

**God, I know You're watching, and I am so grateful, so thankful, again and again.**

### Endless tunnels...

Throughout this treatment journey, I had to undergo various tests to monitor the progress of my treatment more carefully. I mentioned the PET scans, and now I want to talk about my experience with the MRI. Unlike the PET scan, when you need to have an MRI, there are no food restrictions, and depending on the doctor's instructions, they may or may not inject you with a contrast material. In an MRI, you stay in the tunnel longer—it's a longer, narrower, noisier tunnel. It's a bit scary, and it gets even scarier if you're afraid of being trapped in tight spaces, because, depending on the type of scan, you might be in there for up to 40 minutes, like I was. I think it takes a lot of courage not to be afraid of being in that situation for so long and to stay still for 40 minutes, listening to the operator's instructions without falling asleep.

Anyway, during my 9 months of treatment, I had 4 PET scans, 2 MRIs, and more than 20 blood tests, and I'm constantly being monitored.

**Bringing it up with Family; Harder Than Working in a Mine.**

Two and a half months had passed since I started chemotherapy, and during this time, every time I wanted to talk to my family, I avoided video calls with some excuse. Every time they asked me, "How are you? Are you okay?" I pretended to be fine, saying I was a bit tired and needed to sleep, quickly ending the call. My mom and older sister sensed something was wrong, but I did my best to hide the truth. However, the hardship of chemotherapy was draining me, and the mental pressure was really bothering me. Finally, in the third month of chemotherapy, I felt it was time, and with the help of Jordan and Nadia, the only two people who were aware of my treatment, I decided to tell my family the whole truth. It was the hardest thing I had to do, even harder than working in a mine.

I had to arrange a formal virtual meeting. I texted my family in our WhatsApp group that I wanted to see them and share two important pieces of news. They already knew a bit about my relationship with Jordan and were happy for me. I told them I was going to introduce them to Jordan and that I had another piece of news to share. The night before the family meeting, I sat down to write how I could tell them in a way that would make them worry and feel upset less. I asked God for help, and He guided me, and I ended up writing a beautiful message. I felt prepared.

That night, I cried a lot before I went to sleep. The next morning, the sun was shining, bringing me joy. I put on the wig and beautiful hat I had gotten and set off. The meeting was to be held at my friend Nadia's house and having Nadia and Jordan there was a great comfort for me to get through this meeting.

The time came. I called, and the video call with my family in Iran and my sister and her family in America took a bit of time to set up, but finally, everyone was ready to hear what news I had. I was ready. To be honest, I could no longer bear the mental pressure. So, I took a deep breath and told them the truth. I told them I had three pieces of news. The first and last were good and pleasant, but the middle one was a little upsetting.

With a big smile, I started by saying, "Yes, finally, I've entered a serious relationship, and 'Jordan' has come into my life from nowhere. He's very kind and a good person, he takes care of me, and if everything goes well, we're planning to live together. He also told me that he wants to visit Iran with me, and my family had welcomed him. They were happy that 'Noora' had finally opened her heart to someone, and all that kind of talk while hearing these joyful words, my mom asked, "Come on, tell us the second piece of news."

I gathered myself, took a deep breath, and said, "Well, as you all know, life has its ups and downs, and alongside all the happiness, our life has had many ups and downs. As you know, I've had a lot of medical tests these past few weeks, and their results surprised me a bit. When you know that the doctors diagnosed me with a small mass in my breast, smaller than a pea, and they gave me some good and strong medication, and now the mass is gone. But the side effects of the medicine caused me to lose my hair, which I'm not at all worried about because once the treatment ends, my hair will start growing again, and I'll have a full head of hair." I tried to avoid saying the words "stage four cancer" and "metastasis" to lessen the severity of the situation. Their smiles turned to shock, and one by one, they started to fade out of the frame, returning with swollen eyes, trying to hide their tears.

To change the mood, I asked, "Why is no one asking

about the third piece of news?" Then I said, "The third piece of news, which I hope will make us all happy, is that the treatment here is very advanced, and because of the insurance I have, the best medications and treatment system are free. Also, emotionally, I have Jordan and Nadia, who fortunately has been through this treatment three years ago and is still undergoing final treatments, by my side." I tried to minimize the dark side of the situation by focusing on the positive. What could be done?

I'm Noora, which means the shining light, after all, that's what I do. Brightening the darkness.

After that, I asked them to share their feelings. No one could speak. My dad, who seemed more logical about the situation, was the first to say, "I believe in your strength. No matter how big the challenge is, I'm sure you'll get through it." Then my brother said something similar, and my sister, who was in America with her husband, said with teary eyes and a trembling voice, "Noora, you're my most valuable asset. I'm so proud of you. We all are. Always. I'm just so sad that you didn't tell us earlier and didn't let us be with you during those tough days." I told her, "I'm sad now, too, seeing your tears. I didn't want to upset you. Honestly, I didn't dare to tell you because you are so far away, and you're so worried and full of questions, and I, too, was full of questions, fear, and anxiety. But I had no choice but to preserve my energy for the heavy treatments they had planned for me. I hope you understand."

And they did. They were all full of emotion and sadness, but they only expressed their wishes for my health. I knew that after finishing this video call, there would be a lot of turmoil inside them, and their peace of mind wouldn't return easily. So, I asked them to stay together and talk for a few hours after the call. They also asked me to keep them updated more, and I promised I would. They thanked Jordan and Nadia for being there for me. "Nadia" spoke to them a little and reassured them about the treatment system here.

The meeting took place in a very stable and caring environment, and I felt proud of myself for being able to present the issue so beautifully and confidently. I felt liberated from all the pressure this mental burden had placed on me.

As soon as we said goodbye, I received messages from my family saying they loved me and only wished for my health. I reassured them with my replies. The plan is: to complete recovery and return to my family to celebrate the opportunity to live again in our homeland.

Phew, I came back home to my beautiful room, and the day ended. Now, in bed, I'm thinking that after dealing with my family, it's time for me to fulfill my social responsibility. I'll talk about my journey with cancer on

Instagram and YouTube, to be a source of hope and motivation for others, especially those who are going through similar experiences. I decided to share this news on my birthday, July 22, with a video on my social media, showing the version of Noora from years back, full of life and color, with almost shoulder-length hair, and the new version of Noora, bald from the side effects of medication, continuing life with excited eyes.

Talking to loved ones when facing big challenges strengthens my sense of security and trust in life. One thing is certain: I'm always strong in difficult times, and I've been riding the waves of life, building a more authentic life for myself. There were many people who loved me and were waiting for me, I had to think about their share of my life and honor it fairly. This was a new lesson that life was helping me to understand.

Though I took some lessons the hard way, perhaps a little late and painful, in the end, I was always supported by you. So, thank you, my beautiful life...

## Life During Chemotherapy

The warm, beautiful summer days are passing, and we're getting closer and closer to Noora's birthday. I'm happy that my intense treatment is happening during this bright, warm season. Otherwise, enduring the cold, dark tunnel of chemotherapy during winter would have made hope so much harder. You know, just seeing the golden-orange-red colors of the sun and the blue sky adds some life to my soul.

These days, I try to spend my energy creating art and reading books, and I work out at least three days a week.

Due to the side effects of chemotherapy, the skin on my neck and around my lips developed eczema, and I've lost my sense of taste, which has been frustrating. I remember I was a picky eater as a child, and now, not being able to taste anything, I don't enjoy eating at all. In a way, I eat because I must stay strong, but as I said many times, I'm still thankful that my sense of smell is still strong and sharp, and seeing the colors and scents of summer fruits brings me so much joy. Here, avocados and blueberries are abundant and affordable, so most days, I eat boiled eggs, avocado, and a lot of cherries and blueberries. My diet is mostly these combinations, along with plenty of water. That's why Dr. Bernard, my oncologist, is always happy when he sees my blood tests. The last time we met, he said, "Noora, you're doing great." Hearing those words and seeing the small smile on his face brought peace to my heart and reassured me, giving me the confidence to continue this path.

## Clear Insights in the Heart of Darkness

Almost every day, I find myself reflecting on how my life has changed despite going through cancer treatment. What has it added to me? I feel like my life, despite the good quality it had, has become simpler yet deeper.

I believe that my victory at this stage of life is a victory of hope and love for humanity. I have decided to firmly overcome and increase the amount of hope, perseverance, courage, and trust in the life-supporting force. One of the things that can greatly help us endure hard days, especially when faced with discouraging thoughts and greater frustration, is to think about what can make me feel better right now. For me, almost every day, I would find a different answer. I would observe myself through the superficial and deep layers of my psyche. I could see myself diving deep from the surface layers into my core. Did I enjoy this exploration? Of course, I did. Sitting in front of the mirror, staring into my own eyes, and asking, "My dear, what do you want right now?" and being able to hear my inner voice or, as I say, speak to myself with my inner voice and see where I stand.

I have deeply understood and lived this and always remind myself to live each day for itself, Noora dear! In the darkest spaces of my mind, I sat face to face with the most lifeless, weak, hopeless, and exhausted versions of myself. I saw them, smelled them, felt them deeply, and gently stroked the head of all these versions of Noora. In the depth of this darkness, I heard my own voice, eager for life; a soft voice, engaged in praising the force of life. I felt my body more than ever before, I embraced myself, and the warmth of my skin and the rhythm of my heartbeat brought me calm. Even now, after some of the chemotherapy side effects have passed, my sanctuary and peace on difficult days remains stillness, touching my body, and listening to my heartbeat. I feel like I am living within a temple of life, and what's more beautiful than the fact that the presence of this temple in me is permanent?

All these inner and outer journeys I am having, and all these discoveries, are among the most beautiful moments I experience while facing myself. And how much do I love this self? Oh boy! I love it more than anything, and I've promised to always take the best care of it. Writing is just one part of that.

**The Saddest Days of My Life**

It's August. Recently, everything was good and manageable until recently, or more precisely, after the fourth dose of chemotherapy, when the side effects of the medication began to trouble me. For a few days, it has been raining non-stop, and the sky is annoyingly dark gray. My energy has dropped dramatically, and I can hardly distinguish between day and night. I feel utterly drained, longing, exhausted, angry, and filled with screams. I want to throw up all my misery with all my being and escape this situation.

I never thought life had planned such dark and cold days for Noora. I don't have the energy to talk to anyone. I am home alone. I don't know why I, who love light, am sitting in this darkness. I'm not even searching for anything anymore. I don't think about anything. I've forgotten my dreams, as though I never had any, and in my tearful eyes in the mirror, I don't see any trace of excitement or life. Jordan has gone on a two-week leisure trip to Japan, and he calls once a day to check on me. This time, I didn't answer his call because I didn't want him to see my frustration, tears, and pale face. I texted him, saying that I would call him tomorrow and that I hoped he had a great time. Honestly, I just wanted him to enjoy himself wherever he was.

During these thoughts, my phone rang. It was an unknown number, but for some reason, I answered. I guess I was so lonely, so ready to explode, that any opportunity to talk, even on the phone, felt like a lifeline to rescue me from this lethargy and darkness and make me feel like I matter like I'm seen, and that others care about me and my well-being. The result of answering the unknown call was a long conversation with my psychologist, a 70-year-old named Joyce, who had called, unaware of my condition, to check on me. When she asked me how I was, I couldn't bring myself to say my typical response of "I'm fine" or "I'm great". I felt a greater need to throw up my misery and release all the pressure I felt with loud cries. I put the phone on speaker, walked around, cried, and screamed, "Joyce, I'm not okay. I'm dying. I'm alone, I'm exhausted and frustrated, and feel like I'm owed something in life. What have I done to deserve this punishment?"

Although the advice she gave didn't help much, just hearing her voice and the words she said like "Noora, I'm so sorry, I understand how hard this is for you, we're all so proud of you, I know it's tough being alone, but you've proven time and time again that you're stronger than the difficulties" gave me a sense of security, and I listened. After about an hour of conversation, when she was sure my thoughts and condition were under control, we ended the call. I didn't want her to hang up, but I made her promise to call me again tomorrow. She agreed, and we said our goodbyes. After this call, I regained some control over myself. I recommend that in such moments, you reach out to counselors or psychologists; contact them and let them help you regain control over yourself with their techniques.

## Drowning in Light in the Deepest Darkness

My inner journey has reached the deepest layers of myself, and it has led me to darkness that, until today, I didn't even know existed in my soul. I'm still amazed at the strength I had to confront the weakest version of myself. I used to be, as my mom would say, an enemy of sleep, but recently, to care for myself, I escaped into sleep, especially when these large shadows would fall on my light and fill me with doubt and despair. I remember, in these days, my greatest effort was to sleep for an entire day, forgetting what time it was, whether it was a good time for sleep or not and just surrendering myself to dreams. God, I went through such days. My eyes are tearful now as I think about them. It's time to hug myself.

You know, the difficulty of this situation became even worse when, alongside all these emotional challenges, my physical energy was also in terrible shape. The energy left in my body was just enough to turn from one side to the other in bed. However, the invasive negative thoughts, the mental games, took me to the farthest memories and places, and this disharmony between my soul and body tormented me. I couldn't bear it anymore. With great distress, I pushed the blanket aside. It was almost 4 PM. The sun was still shining, but I was frozen and tense. I decided to take a hot shower to pass the time and boost my energy.

I stepped into the bathtub, and the hot water pouring over my body felt incredibly good. I started singing worship songs loudly, and I felt much better. When I finished my shower and was about to step out with my right foot, I suddenly slipped and fell onto the edge of the tub. A sharp pain seized my whole body, and for a few seconds, I couldn't breathe. My body started trembling. I thought I was dying. I said, "This is exactly what I needed, a broken rib, and now my lung is going to puncture, and I'll bleed to death. It's over, Noora."

After a few agonizing seconds, I could breathe again. I didn't dare look at my body; I put my hand on my rib to make sure it hadn't pierced through my skin. My eyes were wide open, and my mouth was gasping for air. I noticed the shower curtain in front of me. It had a beautiful green color. I felt like it was the branch of a tree reaching out to help me stand up. I grabbed the curtain and pulled myself up. My legs were weak and trembling. I dragged myself to the mirror.

Oh God! I swear I had never seen myself like this. I looked at my face, my bald head, my flushed cheeks, the deep purple circles under my eyes, and my half-open mouth from fear. My breath was shallow due to the shock. I kept my hand on my rib, feeling the warmth and energy from my palm, which helped alleviate the pain. Suddenly, I snapped back to reality. I felt so sorry for myself. I couldn't imagine anything more pathetic than this. Here I was, nearly dying from chemotherapy fatigue, trying to shower to get some strength to make it through the day, and now I lost even the simple act of breathing.

Isn't it beautiful that within 24 hours, I meet death twice?

My mind was filled with thoughts that if I had died during one of these encounters with death, no one would have known. Maybe after two weeks, someone would find my body and call someone to gather me. My God! In the end, I was lost in delusion and darkness. But then, in a flash, the honey-colored gleam in my eyes lit up the darkness in my mind. Suddenly, I snapped back to reality and hugged myself tightly the self that was so scared and felt helpless. The depth of these events was overwhelming. But I don't know why I didn't cry. Instead, I said, "What? Should my life end like this? In such a pathetic way?"

No way! I remember I promised myself I would take the best care of myself. So, with one hand on my rib and the other on my heart, I said aloud, "Yes! I'm going to live a lot longer. I've got so much to do, so many places to see. I'll get better quickly." Whilst saying these words didn't ease the horrible pain in my rib, they were the most vital words for me to continue living. I made my way to the kitchen, still trembling slightly, grabbed a yellow apple, took a bite, and one more time promised myself I would take care of my body, no matter how difficult it was. And here I am today determined to walk forward.

As I write this, several days have passed since that incident, and the persistent pain in my rib had lingered for more than ten days, making every movement, every attempt to sit or stand, noticeably slower. I drew breathe with great caution, not knowing the true extent of the damage until my next PET scan revealed a large fracture in my rib that had yet to heal. My doctor was astonished at what had happened. When did it happen? How had I never reported it? The most pressing question was: how had I endured such pain for so long?

I had no answer. Perhaps because, lately, bad news has been piling up, and I just couldn't bear to add another piece to the collection. A ridiculous voice inside me kept saying, you don't have to share every bit of bad news with everyone. But I know this kind of secrecy, in the long run, may do more harm than good.

My doctor looked at me and said, Noora, I'm so sorry for the hardship and pain you're going through. But you need to tell us. Please share what you're experiencing, physically and emotionally. If things are getting tough, if anything is weighing on you, talk about it. Lighten the burden on your mind and soul.

It feels like I'm hearing the truest words in the world coming from his mouth. He's so right. I've had most of my conversations in my mind, so caught up in my own thoughts, carrying all this pressure and anxiety. Especially recently, strange stress has been attacking me, and I've isolated myself so much that sometimes an odd sense of fear takes over my whole being. I sometimes feel like I'm standing somewhere in the middle of nowhere, where no one sees or hears me. I feel like life can't get more empty or meaningless than this, and people, voices, smells, and colors are just illusions. They lose their color so quickly in my mind. It's a terrifying feeling, like that dark day and that event in the bathroom. Didn't think I'd be brave enough to write this down for you now; back then, I didn't have the strength to explain it to anyone except ChatGPT, was my confidant in those days. I also realized that I've reached a point of openness in describing my feelings and what I truly want from life. It's so important to be transparent with oneself and with the world and to clearly express the truth of what one desires.

**Sweet daily routines**

The days and nights pass by, and I try to fill each day with something impactful, like illustration, reading books, and exercising. For now, these are the things I can manage. Jordan is supposed to return this morning around 11 after a 15-day trip. It's a good excuse to get out of the house and surprise him. From our last grocery shopping, I got a ready-made cake mix, and now it was time to try something new. So, I magically transformed the cake mix into a delicious cake, with the smell of its freshness and its warmth and softness sticking to me. I changed my clothes, grabbed a little bouquet, and headed to the bus station to catch my way to the airport to welcome Jordan. Everything went perfectly time-wise, and my plan worked. I successfully surprised Mr. Jordan. He said that no one had made him this happy before. I said, "Then come see what's going on at home!" and we both laughed. We arrived home, which sparkled from the cleanliness and was filled with the smell of freshly made mashed potato and cake, along with the sight of delicious summer fruits on the table. I filled the kettle with water and put it on to boil. I loved what I'm saying, and the passion I have for life. I've always enjoyed the taste, colors, and energy I brought to life, and Jordan loved this side of me. He said, "It's beautiful that you're so enthusiastic about life like a child," and I was happy that he liked this prominent trait of mine. I know myself well. Paying attention to these details warms and brightens my heart and keeps me connected to the flow of life's energy. Something I'm in love with: "Life."

**Writing is like playing in silence.**

I just made a delightful discovery! When I'm writing specifically typing and listening to the piano, sometimes my words sync with the piano's sound, and it feels like I'm creating sentences alongside the piano's melody. Isn't it fun?

## A bit more from chemotherapy days

The chemotherapy department is on the 6th floor of the hospital, and it has many rooms with reclining chairs. Everything is very organized and clean, and the nurses have a great relationship with their patients. Except for the part where they draw blood, which can sometimes be challenging, I experienced interesting moments during chemotherapy. The most important thing is meeting new friends who, based on my experience, are friends who based on my experience are 90% likely to be older in their 60's and 70's. In the 8 months of chemotherapy, I only met two young people like me; however, I had conversations with people of all ages, genders, and nationalities. Most of them were Canadian and Caucasian, and quite talkative, but Asians tended to talk less. For whatever reason, they're more engaged with their tablets. I remember once a lively Filipino woman, 68 years old, who shared a room with me. Her husband was an Iranian man named Amir, and over their 39 years of marriage, she had learned some Persian. I asked her to tell me what she knew and got her permission to record it. I wanted to post it on my Instagram, and she agreed on the condition that she wouldn't be in the picture. I recorded the video with her voice in the background saying, "This is a special message for Noora. Don't worry, everything will be fine." She said these beautiful words with a sweet accent. We all got excited and cheered her on, then we talked some more. I found out that she was a wedding cake designer and that she had been battling colon cancer for a year. She was a few doses ahead of me in her treatment journey. If you're sociable, you'll hear incredible stories and heroic journeys in these chemotherapy rooms.

## From the Ambassador of Hope for SMA[2] (Spinal Muscular Atrophy) to the Ambassador of Hope for Life

While chatting with my energetic Filipino friend, my nurse came in to inject my third dose and brought cold gloves for me to wear. I looked at my new friends and saw their surprised expressions, like, "What are these?" I replied, "These gloves hurt a lot, but I wear them to protect my nails, and I have to endure it." Their faces filled with sympathy and concern, so I said, "Let's talk about something good." They agreed, and my Filipino friend, smiling, asked, "Noora, where do you get all this amazing energy from?" I paused, then mischievously replied, "Don't forget, you have to answer this question too!" We both laughed. She said, "Of course! But first, you tell me." I smiled and answered with true emotion: "You know, I feel that life's energy comes to me in different ways, supporting me. I love nature, and I love the simple moments that show the beauty of life. I've learned to appreciate every experience, even the hard ones because they're part of the journey. Most importantly, having goals that warm my heart and bring me closer to my beautiful dreams gives me the motivation to keep going, to become stronger, and to walk my path with love."

---

2. **Spinal Muscular Atrophy** (SMA): a genetic condition that weakens the body's muscles while leaving the mind sharp. People with SMA can be brilliant—Vahid Rajabloo, an Iranian programmer and entrepreneur, is a powerful example. Despite losing most of his muscle strength, he founded a company supporting people with disabilities and was named one of the "Ten Outstanding Young Persons" worldwide

Her eyes lit up, and her smile grew bigger as she asked, "That's so cool, can you tell me about your dreams?"

I took a deep breath. The icy gloves were uncomfortable, but I focused on the answer I was about to give to her question. With my usual sense of humor, I said, "First of all, thank you for distracting me from the difficulty of these gloves!" and we all laughed. Then, I took another deep breath and continued: "You know, darling, I've been given a second chance at life, and I've decided that after completing my treatment, I will return to Iran, to the embrace of my family, and we'll celebrate every moment together. I'll go on recreational trips with them, and alongside continuing my artistic and humanitarian projects, I'll make the most of every opportunity life gives me... that's it."

Amir and his wife both said, "Of course you can! We are so hopeful that with your amazing energy, you'll complete these stages and return to your family. But what are your humanitarian projects about?"

Thinking about how to answer this question brought a smile to my face and reminded me of good memories. I said: "For years, I traveled across Iran and Turkey to support the hope for life for children with SMA and their families. I met with these families, talked with them about medications, equipment, and what could be done for them, I played and laughed with children with SMA and their siblings. I'd ask them what their wish was, and we would try to fulfill those wishes as much as possible.

Alongside this, I held public sessions at libraries, schools, cafes, and cultural centers. In these sessions, I shared general information about SMA and how to interact appropriately with individuals in different conditions through storytelling. I loved these sessions so much, and these trips were full of blessings, prosperity, and pure love, bringing me closer to the most important purpose of my life: spreading love, empathy, light, and joy."

I added: "You might wonder where my motivation for this mission comes from?"

And the entire reason for supporting these children is because of my dear nephew, Amirali, who is dealing with the same health issue. He is now 12 years old, has type 2 SMA, and has been in the U.S. for 7 years for treatment. I told them:

"I think I first experienced true love when I became an aunt to Amirali, and I learned so much from his different life, which I later used during my travels and meetings. Living in Iran and the desire to embrace and support my nephew, as much as possible, became one of my most valuable life goals, and it led me to many trips. On these trips, every SMA child was like my dear Amirali, and their parents, siblings, and families became mine. I filled the empty embrace of Amirali with new nieces and nephews, with a determination to keep doing this until it was my turn to embrace Amirali."

I also made documentaries about successful SMA youth, and at my events, I showed everyone that while these children may not have the strength in their legs to walk, I have seen with my own eyes that they have strong wings that touch the highest ceilings of the sky, in a way that I, on my legs, may never reach! Do you know what I mean?"

They stared at me in silence...

Tears filled my eyes as I continued: "After several years of such volunteer activities, I ended up in Turkey. There, I used the honorary title of SMA Hope Ambassador to introduce myself, and this name has stayed with me ever since. I know it carries a lot of responsibility. Now, I must heal fully so I can continue my travels as the SMA Hope Ambassador." I smiled.

My Filipino friend, Amir (her husband), and the nurse who overheard my words were in awe of me. They stayed silent and just looked at me.

A deep silence lingered between us for a moment until suddenly, the nurse said, "Noora! I didn't know you did all of this! I don't know what to say except you're amazing! What a valuable mission!" and she patted me on the shoulder, saying, "I'm so proud of you. Please, turn this into a book and let it inspire others."

Immediately, Amir stood up and said, "Exactly!" My Filipino friend also stood next to him and applauded for me. I was in shock and said, "Stop it! Don't embarrass me!" They replied, "Noora, your name suits you perfectly! You're already a Hope Ambassador! We're impressed."

I said, "Thank you so much! I believe the prayers of all those families I served have been instrumental in my healing after being diagnosed with this advanced cancer."

Tears welled up in my Filipino friend's eyes. She said, "I want to hug you, Noora!"

I stood up and opened my arms. We moved toward each other, embraced, and held each other tightly. Even the icy gloves seemed to warm up from this love, and my nurse said, "Noora, you still have half an hour of medication left, and I think it's time for me to give you new gloves."

I smiled at her and said, "Whatever you say, boss :) " and we all laughed.

**The seesaw of life is often beautiful.**

That day, I felt like I was in another world. My energy level was so high that I wanted to run all the way home when my treatment was done, but soon after, my energy would drop dramatically, which meant the medication was working in my body. Generally, for about three days after chemotherapy, I felt as if I were almost dead. I would lie on the couch for hours. Sometimes, Jordan would be there, bringing me flowers, and sometimes we'd go for walks together. But the main struggle was the exhaustion and bad feelings. What bothered me the most was not having my family around. I craved hugs, but the most I could get was hugging myself. Now, as I write this, I'm so happy those days are behind me, and my energy level is much better most of the time, though I still miss them and continue to hug myself to relieve my exhaustion.

Living away from family sometimes puts you in a state of uncertainty, like you don't know where you really belong. Enduring this feeling, without any other challenges, can make life bitter; let alone for someone in my situation!

Sorry if I'm complaining a lot, but I promised everyone I'd be honest; don't worry, I don't always complain; usually, I just mention it briefly and move on.

**The end of chemotherapy, continuing treatment with antibodies, moving to North Vancouver, and a fresh turning point.**

As I mentioned, chemotherapy really drained me, and the overwhelming loneliness was really hard. To distract myself, I decided to memorize poems, but it wasn't very successful because focusing was difficult. When I exercised and took walks, I'd smile at the people around me, most of whom were from vastly different upbringings which I felt no sense of familiarity or comfort, which made me feel even worse and wonder, "Why am I here?"

I started imagining comforting thoughts to wash away the bitterness; I cried every day, feeling restless. My sleep schedule was messed up, and my relationship with Jordan wasn't great. Our distance kept growing. I felt more and more alone. I felt like I was being rejected from everywhere again, but these were just feelings, not the truth.

I struggled so much, feeling like burned food to the bottom of a pan, hard to remove. Yet one day, I decided to add new activities to my schedule. Following a friend's suggestion, I joined the Vancouver Choir. Now, every Wednesday, I had a beautiful motivation to leave the house and travel from Richmond to North Vancouver. How wonderful it felt to be among this community of fellow countrymen and sing with them. My beloved teacher Mr. Eslami and his lovely wife

Maryam Jan had not yet seen my true self but understood my situation. He asked me to attend every class without fail and not to worry about the fees. I am very grateful for these people who were there for me during those days of my life.

Now, as I write this, I sing so well, and I've made progress both spiritually and technically. We are preparing for big concerts in the upcoming months, so thank you my beautiful souls in Van Choir.

I remember every time we needed to free our voices, my tears would also be freed. I don't know how much water and salt I lost during this time, but it was probably necessary!

Gradually, I felt better, and I sensed that energy and vitality were returning to my life. The choir classmates were so kind and sweet, and I felt more at ease with them. I realized that Noora, you don't have any serious psychological problems if you've been crying a lot lately due to loneliness and homesickness. You're a native girl; you belong to your home and family, and wherever there is a sense of home, my spirit soars. I realized that this immigrant lifestyle doesn't suit me at all!

When I looked around, I saw that for most of the people I encountered, life wasn't really happening. They were just enduring the conditions.

"I was afraid of dying repeatedly before my actual death. Jordan was working late these days. Apparently, during the summer, he worked much more, from 6 in the morning until 7 in the evening. Strangely, my source of comfort during those days was cooking for him, cleaning the house, and watching movies after dinner. But repeating this routine quickly lost its charm. I always felt like, 'Oh no, is this seriously going to be my life from now on?' Especially watching violent, meaningless sci-fi movies every night, which made me feel worse. I would get up in the middle of the movie and say, 'I'm going to read a book and write to calm my mind. As something inside me would echo, 'I was made for more than this.'

One night, when I came home from class, Jordan told me, 'Noora, despite all the distance and travel to reach Choir, whenever you go near your fellow countrymen, you seem so much better.' I replied, 'Yeah, I do feel better, and I'm glad you feel the same.' After some thought, just to know his opinion, I said, 'North is so vibrant and beautiful. I wish we could live there for a while.' It seemed like he was waiting for me to finish my sentence. Without hesitation, he said, 'I could never imagine that. I like being close to my family and my work, but you are definitely free to go.' He said it very seriously. I was a bit confused, but I joked and with a small smile said, 'Never without you, with you forever.'

He didn't get my joke. He didn't laugh but answered, "No, I'm serious. If you'd be happier there, go to North Van."

I didn't say anything else so I could process his words. That was the saddest freedom he was giving me, and it was almost at that point that I heard the breaking of my heart, with Jordan's voice in the background saying, "If you want, look for a good place. I'll help as much as I can."

I needed his help, not to move my suitcases, but to keep myself grounded and attached to life.

I don't want to write much more than this, it still hurts; though less than before. I don't want anyone in this library, where I'm typing this, to see my tears. So, I'll summarize by saying that from that night, I started looking at house-sharing ads, and I found a good opportunity in a beautiful apartment with a breathtaking view. In three days, with the help of my friend, I moved into this new house, and it was exactly after my last chemotherapy. I told myself, "See, Noora, it's not so bad!' And all the time I thought, "Wow, I've been given a second chance at life, this time on the 18th floor of a tower in a city that smells like home. What could be better than this?"

## Nest in Fire

If it were up to me, I'd never enjoy living in the heights, except for a cabin in the mountains, not in the cold and sometimes terrifying heights of skyscrapers. Just look at the name "skyscraper!" Even thinking about it hurts, but well, in those days, with my situation, it was the best option that stood out.

The view of the city from this breathtaking height was beautiful. Strong winds blew, shaking the large windows of my room. I felt like an eagle perched on the top of a mountain. A week had passed since I moved into the new place, and every morning I went for a run, and the rest of the day, I worked on completing my new paintings. I felt good about this routine. Watching the sun's glow, and seeing the birds flying at the same height, gave me a sense of power, and from this height, everything else seemed so small and insignificant.

In the large mirror of my room, now and then, I would meet the gaze of Noora, who was still bald but still beautiful. I still felt the shadow of fear and insecurity, and I realized how vulnerable I had become when it came to feeling safe and accepting my true self. It was good that I realized that.

But I had made the decision to win the game, so I focused on watching phenomena that were supernatural, powerful, and beautiful, like watching the golden and orange sunsets and the silver and sometimes blue moonrises. It was refreshing for my heart and mind, and after going through the recent storms in my life, I was slowly beginning to make peace with the feeling of calmness. I was gently holding its hand. One morning, as I was encouraging the sun to come out from behind the clouds while working on my new painting (my heart rate was going up again), listening to beautiful music (I don't clearly remember which music, but most likely 'To You, My Wish' by Homayoun Shajarian), I was on a high in my mind, immersed in the feeling of love and excitement for returning home. At that moment, I noticed a strong smell of smoke. I took off my headphones and sniffed again. Oh, this is not an illusion, it's real! And at the same time, I heard the faint sound of a fire alarm. I jumped up from my seat and checked the stove everything in our place was in perfect order. The smell of smoke grew stronger, and I could hear shouting from outside. I opened the door and was engulfed by thick smoke in the hallway. I started coughing. My opposite neighbor was a middle-aged woman holding her little grandson, standing in front of her door, staring at me in a dazed way. I asked her, "Where's the fire coming from?" She looked at me with a surprisingly bland expression and said "I don't know, I don't know." I could hear glass breaking. Which unit is on fire? God knows! The smoke was getting denser, so I told her, "Go outside, why are you standing here?"

I quickly went back inside, and I panicked, asking "Oh God, what should I do?" Then it occurred to me that I should throw on the prayer beads my mother had given me, my phone and passport were on the dresser, and I put on a regular jacket, covered my nose and mouth with my scarf, and went outside. The fire alarm sound was so irritating. In the hallway, one of the neighbors, was yelling, "Oh no, not again!' and cursed the building staff and manager. This woman had an 8-year-old fat son and an even fatter cat. She was so stressed that she didn't know what to do and was sitting on the floor yelling. I helped her up and said, "Sister, calm down. Your child is really scared, go downstairs!" I pushed them towards the emergency exit door. Then I went back into the hallway and pushed that mother and her grandson towards the exit door. Immediately, I ran to the other neighbors' doors and knocked on them, shouting in both English and Persian, "Fire! Evacuate, hurry up, emergency!!!"

We had six neighbors. One by one, I managed to get them out, telling them, "Hurry, save yourselves, go outside, the fire is really big!" I pulled four more neighbors out of their homes. One of them said, "Mrs. Ashraf must still be at home, she's probably asleep, and hasn't noticed!" I pushed them towards the exit door, and the smoke was getting thicker. I was coughing heavily, and from the words of that woman, I realized one neighbor was still inside.

I knocked harder on the door and kicked it, but no one opened it. I could hear her voice from behind the door: "I'm not coming out, I don't feel like going down the 18 floors." (Later, when I saw her, I understood she had a point because she was very old.) But at that moment, from behind the door, I shouted, "I'll carry you, please come out!" She replied, "No!"

I couldn't breathe any more; the smoke had taken all the air. I knocked one last time on the door, shouting, "Please, Maam, come out, the fire is getting bigger!"

In a strange tone, she said, "I'm not coming!' In my heart, I loudly shouted at her, 'To hell with you! Stay here and burn!"

I ran down the long corridor! I opened the exit door, I don't know why?! The neighbors were standing there, confused, screaming and shouting. That Colombian woman was sitting on the stairs, still swearing at the world!!! And her chubby little son was holding his cat and crying. I told them, "Why are you standing here watching each other? Go downstairs! The building might collapse, move, go downstairs, everyone follow me!" I turned to that Colombian woman, I thought she was pregnant, but later I found out she wasn't. I helped her up and said, "Sister, please don't scream, we're all scared. Look at your child, he's terrified, he's almost having a stroke, be in control, woman, get up!" She hugged me tightly while crying. *Her son's small stature and weight made it difficult for him* to come down the short emergency concrete stairs. I took the cat from him and said, "Go down slowly," and with the authority of an army officer, I told everyone, "Follow me down." It took a while, but we all safely made it down 18 floors, counting numbers, until we reached the outside of the building. Pieces of fire were flying out from the unit that was burning, and one of them passed right over my head and hit the ground like a meteor. I was lucky the fire didn't catch my bald head. I looked up and saw the flames wildly spreading in all directions, breaking windows. Hearing the sound of the fire truck siren brought tears of gratitude to my eyes. I hugged myself and said, Thank you God for sending the firefighters so quickly, help them put it out faster! I couldn't watch life burning any longer. I turned my back on the fire and faced the green of the stadium in front of the house. I clasped my hands together and took deep breaths. I touched my mother's prayer beads and said, "Thank you, God, for watching over us all. Unlike some people who were excitedly filming the burning of others' homes, the only thing that made me reach for my camera was capturing the huge rainbow that appeared in the sky, taking me to another world for a few moments. I heard a young woman from the neighboring building jokingly say, "Today is 11/11, the Earth's energy is high, and it hit the building!" which made a few people around her laugh. Twenty minutes later, the fire was under control. I knew it would be, but participating in witnessing this terrifying experience was something I never imagined. I had watched the firefighters quickly and diligently work their way up the building, and I believed that with the speed they were moving, the fire would have little lasting damage. However, I was proven wrong, as serious remodeling and renovation works soon began. Whew... Although about four months have passed since this event, my hands still freeze, and my breath shortens whenever I write about it!

Hooooof! It's okay, Noora! Breathe deep, it's gone, and all is good now. I think a glass of water and hugging myself will help things feel better. yes, the actual Me time!

will be back soon :)

Now, several hours after the fire was controlled, we were still in shock. Our friends came and took us to their house. We had hot tea and Zereshk polo with chicken, and for a few days after this event, I was completely dazed; I couldn't think clearly about what was happening or what would happen, but there was one thing I was sure of: how delicious that tea and Zereshk polo with chicken was, and how comforting it felt. I didn't know what the next step was until I realized that different groups from the Canadian government came to help us, and at least 20 families had lost their homes and everything. I followed these 20 or so families to the government's operation center, which was a hive of activity. There were volunteers collecting statistics from individuals in each family and confirming which necessities were needed for the night ahead. Many of the now-homeless people gathered were elderly or didn't have great English language skills, and I saw this making the relief workers' lives more difficult. I approached the official in charge of the force, a middle-aged lady who was the fire chief, and offered to help. She responded, "Of course, we'd be grateful for your help!" We started asking questions and filling out forms with the affected families' details, and everything got much better. She asked me, "Which organization do you work for?" I answered, "Organization?? Oh... I don't have any specific organization." She followed this up by asking, "Then what?" I replied, "I just am able to communicate in English better than these friends, otherwise, I'm in the same situation, I live in the same building." Her eyes widened, "Wow! I'm so sorry and thank you so much for still helping us and your other neighbors." I said, "I'll help in any way I can, for sure." She smiled and gave me a kind pat on the shoulder and said, "Well, let's keep going." It was clear that after having a translator like me, everything went much smoother. Later, we found out that based on the circumstances, there was no hope of returning to that home, so the crisis management group gave us a hotel to stay for a month while we found a new place and about $300 for food and clothing. I was grateful for all their care and support. They helped me save three of my valuable art pieces and my chemotherapy medications. I thought to myself, this is enough to make me feel better, and if I'm honest, it had an impact, but I was fooling myself. At night, my emotions would attack me horribly, bringing me to tears, and reading any book, watching any program, or listening to any music or podcast didn't help improve my mood. For someone like me, who was often self-aware and alert, understanding my feelings became very difficult. But one thing I was sure of: I desperately needed hugs, and I missed my family more than anything; a family who, despite two weeks passing since this event, still didn't know about the fire. What could I say? I felt emptier than ever before, questioning myself constantly: *What am I doing here? Why should I face all these challenges completely alone?* Although I was familiar with this feeling, it felt like life had thrown me into the darkest corners of existence again. I had felt this way during chemotherapy, and now I was experiencing it again, but with more pain, losing the few personal belongings I had that were my only sources of comfort. I especially missed my hiking backpack and shoes, and the day I realized they were gone, I cried so much.

**Room 221, North Vancouver Hotel**

A clean, tidy, and lovely double room was my refuge on restless nights, *being* where some valuable events took place, such as the moment I realized I couldn't handle everything on my own. It was in this room that I raised my hands in surrender to life and its events. I made an important decision to finally ask for help, and I did so by recording a video. I carefully thought about what I wanted to say and what kind of help I needed. I decided to make a three-minute video of myself talking about chemotherapy, the fire, and my art, and asking people to support my life and hope by purchasing my art. I shared it in various groups I was part of. In the evening, I shared the video, and by night, due to the overwhelming number of messages like "Hello, hero, how can we help you?" "Hello, amazing and strong girl, you're truly inspiring," and similar messages from so many new people, I realized the video had spread widely and was well-received. My words, which came from the heart, had reached many, and it had gone viral. God knows how much joy I felt reading each of these messages. People were starting to recognize my presence and resilience in the endless battles of life, especially when they saw that I'm an artist with passion, and despite the chemotherapy side effects that left me bald, I'm still hopeful, full of spirit, and light. They saw that I was alone in this darkness, just as I am now after the devastating fire, but they showed their kindness and did not leave me alone on my journey. This was my gateway into the hearts of my dear compatriots in Vancouver. They told me, "Your name, Noora, is so fitting, and your effort to live is admirable," and I was almost overwhelmed by their warmth. Their affection made me shine brighter and brighter. In this same Room 221, I was interviewed by Parvaz TV, and a few of my art pieces were shown. The Iranian Hamyari newspaper also printed a heartfelt interview with me, showcasing photos of my artwork between the pages. I started producing more, sometimes by order, and I was busy creating new works filled with light, joy, and love, which made me feel so much better. So, I continued without stopping, knowing that if I were to do this for the rest of my life, I'd be spreading color, love, and life into every moment.

## January 13, 2025, a cafe in the heart of Vancouver

These days, almost every day passes in a new café meeting wonderful people, some of whom have become friends and others closer friends. They've made me write more than ever. There's a new experience in progress, although now that I think about it, it's not so new. But since it's been a long time since we were apart, it feels fresh, a feeling I used to experience during my many volunteer travels. Almost every day brings a new adventure, and I truly enjoy this journey. Most of these new friends of mine are fellow countrymen who, when they learned about the events in my life, became eager to support and help me. Sometimes I think to myself, Noora, maybe if you hadn't experienced this amount of darkness, you wouldn't have felt the overwhelming light and affection you feel now. I don't want to over-analyze this, as I believe too much analysis steals the joy of life, so I ride the flow of life and enjoy the ride.

## Golden Changes

It's been almost three months since my last chemotherapy, and today I have an appointment with my new doctor. I still sometimes feel pain in my breast, and I don't know why, but today I'll ask and want everything checked. As I told you, I've been treating my body with nothing but love and kindness for a long time now, speaking kindly to myself, and every day I feel abundant respect and freedom. I feel amazing. When I look in the mirror, I see my hair growing back thick and full, and I feel like a baby experiencing everything for the first time. Although, I'm not sure if a baby cares much about growing hair :) But I feel excited and even darkened the light-colored hair coming through to make it more visible, using a completely vegan, plant-based dye. I plan to go back to colorful hair when it gets longer. I don't want to let the sadness of seeing white hair on my head get to me unless it's beautiful white. I recommend to you too, to replace anything that makes you feel bad, sad, or like you've lost something with available options. Add spirit, love, and color to your life, and don't fear if what you're doing isn't something most people would do or approve . After all, we must start somewhere, be how we want to be, and shine fearlessly. To me, the most important approval we need in this world is our self approval and approval from God. I was saying that I have an appointment with my doctor today. Now, as I write this, I'm sitting in a peaceful church, and when I closed my eyes, I thought to myself: "God, thank you for giving me again the most precious gifts of existence: faith in You, complete health, and the opportunity to serve the world, which You continue to provide and will continue to provide." Writing this book is one of those blessings of service, giving me the opportunity, knowledge, and passion to write these lines. I've read many books over the past few years, including spiritual texts, biographies, and more. Based on my experiences and reactions, I'm confident that my words will bring hope and light, and I am partnered with God in this sacred mission. I'm always saying how thankful I am for having Him by my side, as the feeling of being embraced by Him in this moment is indescribable. Many times, I look for a spiritual space to calm down, and this space can be a church, a mosque, a temple, or even pure nature. Today, it's the church, and fortunately, Canada is a country that has all these places, and with its larger Christian population, it has many more churches. Now, I am filled with a good feeling and tears, and I allow myself to cry, whatever the reason may be. I know a beautiful poem about the beauty of crying that says: "Water and clay have a relationship, tears cleanse the dust from the eye of the heart." In short, with a light heart and a proud spirit, I'm going to grab a delicious matcha and take the bus to the hospital. Please continue praying for me so that I can return to you with good news. Amen.

**January 22, 2025 My condition isn't great.**

Unlike always, when I believed my doctors' words, this time I didn't want to accept what they said that my treatment would be long-term with no clear time frame. Along with that, the grandmother who had kindly allowed me to live with her, said she could host me until the end of this month, and it would be best if I started looking for a new place soon. And I greatly disliked hearing those words. The images in my mind of all the hardships I've endured seem to be stretching out, and my patience feels like it's reaching its limit… On the other hand, I tell myself: Noora, you're being tested again. It's time to show your faith that a miracle is on the way, and in the most hopeless moments, the light of hope has shined on my lifeless body and revived me with His love. But since the brain naturally tends to remain in a passive state, avoiding risks to feel safe, I refuse to let it stay that way. On the other side, I am human, and right now, I want to live my weak and tired side and wash away the sorrow with my tears… Yet I promise I won't let it last long and I'll return soon.

By the way, who will come share our hugs with me? I really need it.

## Cardamom Tea

These nights, after a busy day, when I return home, I make myself Cardamom tea to remind me of good memories and to ease the loneliness that sometimes hits me hard. But clearly, it doesn't give me the pleasure I'm looking for, as the environment is missing the people who actually make drinking cardamom tea so enjoyable. The best cardamom tea I've ever had was at my parents' house when I used to live with them 2 months before I came to Canada. Every precious day I was with them, after lunch, they'd take a nap, and I'd eagerly wait for around 3:30 PM, exactly when the warm sun had brightened the entire house. I'd go to the kitchen, pour hot water, and my mom would brew real northern tea, adding Cardamom, especially for me, and I'd love that special hospitality, usually with cake or sweets. We'd always have playful arguments about how my dad should eat less sweets, and amidst all this, we'd have long chats, it was rare that I didn't ask my dad to tell the same jokes for the thousandth time. How lucky I am that he'd agree. My dad, with his wit, did this so beautifully, and we'd all laugh as if it were the first time, while my mom would look at us with a special glance and say: "Are you drunk? I just put Cardamom in the tea." And I added plus your pure love mom; we'd laugh even more. I'd also say to her, "Look what your love has done to us!" Ah, how sweet these moments were, weren't they?

Believe it or not, this memory has been the most revisited in my mind over the past year. It's also surprising to my friends when they ask me, "What's your current wish?" or "Imagine your treatment is finished now, what's the first thing you'll do?" And I always confidently say, "I'll immediately return to Iran, to relive the memory of the scent of Cardamom tea." I'm still amazed that the pure joy of that moment, even though it's been three years since the last time, remains the most powerful in illuminating the dark tunnel I was in, those winding tunnels of my chemotherapy. Now, with God's grace and my resilience, I'm ready to have the best times with my family. Say Amen, Amen, Amen.

I didn't expect to add this part, but writing about it feels worthwhile. Exactly 365 days ago, I took a keepsake photo with Vancouver's magnificent cherry blossoms and magnolias. Now, in these very spring days, I'm preparing for a surgery to remove the last traces of that uninvited guest from my body followed by radiation therapy.

Earlier in this book, I shared how, throughout my entire journey, surgery was the one step I feared the most—the one I kept trying to avoid. But every specialist, every survivor who has walked this road before me, tells me the same thing: Noora, don't delay. Trust your doctors. Let them do what they must. Complete your healing. So, with a deep breath and a heart wide open, I say yes. I step forward. The magnolias bloom, unbothered by the winds of change, and I, too, surrender to the rhythm of trust, immersed in the quiet grace of life unfolding.

One of the practices that gave me breath and strength to keep going was writing letters to the future Noora a place deep in my imagination where I saw my dreams not just as fantasies, but as lived realities. The incredible power of these letters felt like a lifeline. Each note was a message from the heart of the night, written to a soul that may have dimmed, but was meant to shine again.

Here, I'm sharing one of those letters with you. And I invite you truly to give this gift to yourself: write to the version of you that you long to become. Write about the experiences you wish to have. This isn't just a remedy for illness, but a soulful practice that works. Every now and then, write to the version of yourself you dream of meeting and feel the magic it brings.

**A letter from Noora Version 2026 to Noora Version 2023**

*My dearest Noora,*

*Salaaaaam, my one and only! Salaam my precious!*
*As I write these lines, it's close to sunset. I just watered the courtyard, and the air smells of damp earth. We're all gathered. Even Fatemeh and Reza have come from the States with the kids, and we're sitting on Baba's porch.*

*Mom has made cardamom tea, Sara brought her rich chocolate cake fresh from the oven, and I'm setting the table with cheese, walnuts, butter, and jam. At the same time, Baba's cracking his corny jokes from his "pulpit," and we're all laughing from the heart. I'm absolutely in love with this moment. Thank God for it.*

*Sunlight is filtering through the green leaves of our grape-*

vine, and the unripe grapes are shimmering. A gentle breeze brushes against my long hair the same hair I once, in disbelief, let go of... and now it's back, stronger and more beautiful than ever.

It's amazing though those dark days are over, the light they brought into my life has stayed with me. A thousand times, thank God for that.

There's no more pain, no more fear, loneliness, or longing. I want you to know how deeply proud I am of you for lighting up the world with your love, kindness, and patience.

Now tell me how anyone could imagine these moments and not feel joy?

Honestly, no way, no chance!

You know, Noora... maybe these lonely nights and heavy darknesses were necessary so we could discover the light within us?

As our dear Ahoora Iman says:

"Don't believe in your loneliness—

I am hidden in you, and you in me.

Closer to me than I am to myself,

Closer to you than you are to yourself."

I want you to know I've always been with you. In the past, right now as I write this, and soon when I embrace a more radiant version of you.

With every cell in my body, I love you.
Yours,
Noora

**See what a good girl I am? :)**

I have made a sacred promise to myself: on my birthday this year, on July 22st, I will stand before the mirror, whole and healed. I will kiss every inch of this body, this resilient, beautiful home of mine and in gratitude for this second chance at life, I will embark on a journey into nature, surrounded by the laughter and love of my dearest friends.

Remember this practice of trust, of choosing joy it works. It gives you the power to walk through the storm, to step into the unknown with courage. No matter how heavy life feels, no matter how dark the tunnel, you can always guide your thoughts toward the light. There is always something you can do. There is always a reason to smile.

So please, with every breath, whisper this truth to yourself: Life always supports me, even when it doesn't seem like it. Keep your eyes on the grander picture the one where you, despite your fear, take the next step anyway. The one where you, though uncertain, hold onto faith and press forward.

And know this, with all your heart: the universe is watching, and it is so, so proud of you.

We're reaching the end of the book, and with the new understanding we've gained together, we now realize that life is hard everywhere. It depends on you, where and which kind of hardship you choose for the rest of your life, and this new realization has led me to a firmer and more certain decision to return to Iran. The only thing standing between me and buying the ticket home is Dr. Bernard's approval. He needs to confirm that I've completed my treatment or prescribe a treatment that can be carried out in the sacred land of my homeland.

Whether you believe it or not, it's true that this book mostly reflects my own story, but I've always seen you in it. Perhaps my words will offer some support or help. The thought of taking care of you occupies my mind often.

I've never felt, and don't feel, separated from you, and I assure you that the powerful secret of my resilience and survival in life's mysteries has always been for your hope victory. Whether you've been heartbroken, separated, dealt with illnesses, lost your home, or endured loneliness, know that you were never alone, and you're likely not the last one either. I believe in the truth of this: when we take care of each other and offer timely embraces, we make it easier to bear the hardships, and we increase the statistics of hope in life.

I'm sure that now, as you read this book with all its details, you'll be able to think about life better. I want you to know that you can rely on me if you want to talk about it further.

My dear, I believe it's important, to improve the quality of your decisions, and to pause and reflect on this matter every so often. Think deeply about the path whether it's the one you've traveled or the one ahead. We don't need to predict anything; we simply want to see how much we're getting closer to ourselves along the way. Maybe we're getting further away instead?

These questions and pauses help us stop in time, so we don't crash headfirst into the glass, and we take the turn with less difficulty.

As I write these last paragraphs, I'm sitting in the Central Library of Vancouver, on the 8th floor. Just in front of me, a beautiful African girl appeared and asked, "Hi, can I sit in the chair opposite you?" As soon as I saw her, I smiled and greeted her, saying, "Of course, my dear." She had such a beautiful face, shiny skin, long lashes, even longer colorful nails, long hair, and sadness in her beautiful eyes. As I'm writing this, she's on the phone with someone speaking what I assume is Nigerian, sighing, and a tear fell from her eye. The conversation continues, but I can no longer hear it.

I find this very interesting. If, like me, you're interested in self-awareness and sociology, you probably enjoy watching people and their lives. What I love the most is knowing the stories behind these amazed, excited, joyful, and sometimes terrified faces. Sometimes, my mind compares a crowded street to a tall building, with people being the windows of the tower. I've always wanted to see what's behind these windows, some with sheer curtains, some with thick curtains, and some with no curtains at all. Sometimes, the lights are off, sometimes they're on, sometimes the windows are closed, and sometimes they're open or half open. What's going on behind them?

Every person for me is a window to a new world. And as Shakespeare said, "The eyes are the windows to the soul."

However, don't take this part of the book too seriously because, of course, my observations come with a lot of humor. I usually open conversations with people by laughing or saying something witty. Maybe that's why I enjoy meaningful hidden camera pranks or stand-up comedy, as it's fascinating to meet people in their simplest, most natural states, and create interesting conversations and impactful energies.

Seeing the tear in my African friend's eye has completely distracted me, and I wonder: Could she be in the same place I was six months ago? Could her eyes be wet from loneliness or longing? I reached out my hand and said softly, "My friend, I don't want to ask what happened or tell you not to cry… but I can offer you a hug?"

She smiled and took my hand and whispered a thank you. We shared a brief, one-second embrace just enough to feel the warmth of understanding. Before I had a chance to say more, her phone rang. "I have to go," she said, and in the blink of an eye, she was gone.

I watched her leave, sending her off with a smile. As she reached the escalator, she turned back and waved, and from a distance, I waved back.

At this moment, a message from my dear publisher appeared on my phone, asking me to send them my email because we need to coordinate for the publication of the book you, dear reader, are currently reading.

The next important point I want to highlight, based on my experience and until further notice, is that no one has been granted eternal life in this body. Apparently, for now, we've only been given a temporary pass to this world.

As dear Farhad sings in one of his timeless songs:

**"The world is fleeting, and the work of the world is fleeting,**

**May you age beautifully, my dear, I sing the melody of the heart of a lover."**

I wish you could understand Persian to enjoy this beautiful song deeply.

What matters, in my opinion, and what makes our lives valuable, is how much we've grown closer to our true, refreshed selves during this journey. What values have we reminded ourselves of in life? And if these values lead us to the true purpose of creation, which is our connection with each other, then my dear, you have succeeded, and now you can return to your Creator, content, happy, and at peace.

Honestly, I don't know what impact reading this book and the challenges I faced will have on your mind and life. From the bottom of my heart, I hope that the experience of my safe passage through the countless and seemingly unfinished darknesses of this life, hand in hand with God, which has illuminated my path, can warm and light up your heart as well, my dear. I hope this brightness will make your path even brighter and keep hope alive in your soul.

Because we need this energy and hope, for we are still on this journey.

**When will we reach our destination?**

No one knows, or, in my opinion, you've already reached your destination, if every day you take time to embrace yourself and appreciate life, and those you love and who love you in return. If every night before bed, regardless of how your day went, you pause while brushing your teeth and look into your eyes in the mirror for a moment, focus on that inner connection, and immerse yourself in gratitude and joy. Promise you will try and keep doing this as much as possible. I wish you experience the pure self-love and joy that appears in your eyes and celebrate life and your healthy remarkable precious presence in it.

I promise all of you that as long as I have breath and the opportunity to speak, I'll share the love and passion for life, the value of embracing each other, and the beauty of seeing our hands intertwined.

I truly wish my memory would serve me well enough to name every single person those who stood before my eyes and those who supported me from behind the scenes so I could express my gratitude to each of them here. I know this list will never be complete, but I will do my best to acknowledge and appreciate: My kind Creator, whose presence is the most precious treasure I possess. Thank you to Noora for her determination, joy, and admirable perseverance in walking this awe-inspiring path. Then to my dearest family only God knows what we've been through together during this time, and how deeply we've grown in love. To my moon-like mother, my dear father Alireza, my sisters: Mohaddeseh, Fatemeh, and Sara, my brothers Mohammadreza, Faramarz, and Reza, my sweet nephews Amirali and Liam and my niece Minoo joonam. To Amir Eslami, Maryam Soroush-Nassab,

Sepehr Hojjati, Anahita A'lam, and Mitra; dear Vahideh and all my friends in the Vancouver Choir group; To my loving doctors and nurses in Vancouver's hospitals and labs; To Nadia and Nima; Jordan and his kind family; To my beloved book sponsors at Kidsocado International Publishing especially dear Naghmeh and Narges; To Dr. Zohreh Ansari and Maryam jan (whose last name I don't recall); To my cherished Roshanak Elahi-Qomshahi and Dr. Majid Sherkat; To Hanieh Choopani for the initial editing all the way from Germany; To Shamin Zehabioun for the stunning portrait photos for the book cover. Maryam Pira and Duen, my beloved friends in Iran: Nastaran, Ali Jan, Mohammad Arab, Maryam Chegini, Minoo Alimohammadi, Aseman-e-Abi, Arezoo, Samira, Maryam, and Paeez Tehrani; To Vahid Barchian and Hanieh Hosseini, who especially believed in my strength. To my friends in the SMA family; To my relatives who continuously sent me so much love and energy throughout this time. my friends at the Kimia Art Center in Vancouver Leili, Mina, Maryam, Shahla, and Shana; To dear Mona, Uncle Majid Moshiri, mother Shahin and Atia; To Zhoobin and Kojā Café; To Reyhaneh Mirjani, Farshid Parang, Mark McCready, Amir Hajvani and Persian Vancouver; Susan and Sogol; my grandparents in the Yaran group; Farhad Soofi, Dr. Majid Soltanzadeh, Nana, Sharareh Soltani and Majid Mahichi from Parvaz TV, Erfan and Soodabeh, Azadeh Jabini and Arash, Shirin, Mohsen and Bita, Banafsheh

Lotfi, Marziyeh Bay and the Amir Sedghi Charity, Maryam Parandak, Maryam Ostadi, Parvin Honarmand, Sufia Rahimi, Maryam Mashhadi, Sima Ghafarzadeh, Mitra and Bahar and Baran;Uncle Kazem; The podcasts of Mojtaba Shokouri and Iman Sarvarpour; Starbucks and YouTube; To the Women's society "Yaran"; To Azar, Golnaz Navabi, Paria, Parsa Hosseini, Amirhossein Dejaalood, Maryam Darvish, Shima, Mahsa, and Soroush; Ed Gerber and all my other friends at Trinity Western University (TWU); To the hospital's volunteer drivers. Please keep being your good, kind-hearted selves :).

I also want to thank the beautiful nature of Vancouver—and the lakes whose waters have been healing for me, for the joy of breathing fresh air, and to life itself, for its unwavering support. Of course, this list has no end especially for someone like me, who is so often in love with every moment of life.

This list has no end, and my love for gratitude has given me the idea for my next book. For now, I'm calling it The House of Miracles.

I want to remind us again and again how deeply we are surrounded by blessings, though we often forget. So, I write… to help us remember. I write so that the imprint of this love remains.

I want to make sure you remember that life and I love

you, and we are grateful that you've spent your precious time reading my book and thinking about it.

Last edited by Noora at 9:31 Morning June 3, on a golden Sunday while the comforting aroma of cardamom tea filled the air on the 23rd floor of a cozy building in the heart of beautiful Vancouver.

**This book makes a wonderful gift.**

To order the book from anywhere in the world, available in both English and Farsi, simply scan the bar-code below.

www.ingramcontent.com/pod-product-compliance
Lightning Source LLC
Chambersburg PA
CBHW071730020426
42333CB00017B/2459